History on
the Couch

History on the Couch

Essays in History and
Psychoanalysis

EDITED BY

*Joy Damousi and
Robert Reynolds*

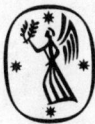

MELBOURNE UNIVERSITY PRESS

MELBOURNE UNIVERSITY PRESS
An imprint of Melbourne University Publishing (MUP Ltd)
PO Box 1167, Carlton, Victoria 3053, Australia
mup-info@unimelb.edu.au
www.mup.com.au

First published 2003
Text © Joy Damousi and Robert Reynolds 2003
Design and typography © Melbourne University Publishing (MUP Ltd) 2003

Typeset in Meridien 10 point by Syarikat Seng Teik Sdn Bhd
Malaysia
Printed inAustralia by McPherson's Printing Group

National Library of Australia Cataloguing-in-Publication entry

History on the couch: essays in history and psychoanalysis.

Bibliography.
Includes index.
ISBN 0 522 85057 X.

1. Psychohistory. 2. Psychohistory—Case studies. I. Damousi, Joy, 1961–.
II. Reynolds, Robert, 1965–.
901.9

Contents

Contributors

Bain Attwood is a Senior Research Fellow at the Centre for Cross-Cultural Research at the Australian National University. He has published widely on the history of relations between Aboriginal and settler Australians. His most recent book is *Rights for Aborigines* (Allen & Unwin, 2003).

John Cash is Deputy Director of the Ashworth Program in Social Theory at The University of Melbourne and an editor of the international journal *Critical Horizons*. He was an undergraduate at the University of Melbourne and took his doctorate in political science at Yale University, concentrating on political psychology and social and political theory. His research focuses on the political/cultural unconscious and its centrality to the organisation of subjectivities and social and political relations.

Catharine Coleborne is the co-editor (with Diane Kirkby) of *Law, History, Colonialism: The Reach of Empire* (Manchester University Press, 2001) and the co-editor (with Dolly MacKinnon) of *'Madness' in Australia: Histories, Heritage and the Asylum* (University of Queensland Press, forthcoming). She has published work on the history of madness in Australia in these and in several other collections, including *Sex, Power and Justice*, *Forging Identities*, and in Roy Porter and David Wright's collection of international essays on the confinement of the insane (Cambridge University Press, forthcoming). Her current work considers psychiatry in the museum and the construction of psychiatric histories in Australia and New Zealand. She lectures in history at the University of Waikato, New Zealand.

Judith Brett teaches politics at La Trobe University. She is the author of *Robert Menzies' Forgotten People* (Macmillan, 1992) and editor of *Political Lives* (Allen & Unwin, 1997) a collection of psychobiographical essays on political leaders.

Joy Damousi is an Associate Professor in the Department of History at the University of Melbourne. Her recent work includes *The Labour of Loss: Mourning, Memory and Wartime Bereavement in Australia* (Cambridge, 1999) and *Living With the Aftermath: Trauma, Nostalgia and Grief in Post-war Australia* (Cambridge, 2001). She is currently writing *Freud in the Antipodes*, a history of psychoanalysis in Australia.

Miriam Dixson trained in history at the University of Melbourne, completed a PhD at the Australian National University, and is now an Honorary Fellow at the University of New England in Armidale, NSW. Her study of women and identity, *The Real Matilda*, is an Australian feminist history classic, with a first edition in 1976 and a fourth in 1999. Her book *The Imaginary Australian* draws on object relations and was also published in 1999. It addresses some of the defining issues of a new century—globalisation, localism and the inner life, identity, ideology and the social imaginary.

Esther Faye is a Lacanian psychoanalyst who also teaches in the Department of History at the University of Melbourne in the areas of Holocaust memory and history. She has published a number of articles and chapters on the unconscious memories of 'the Jewish second generation' in Australia, and she is currently working on a book titled *Displaced Encounters with the Holocaust*.

Christopher E. Forth is a senior lecturer in history at the Australian National University. He is the author of *Zarathustra in Paris: The Nietzsche Vogue in France, 1891–1918* (2001) and *Conquering Virility: The Dreyfus Affair and the Crisis of French Manhood* (forthcoming). He is currently writing a history the male body in the Western world.

Rose Lucas teaches in the School of Literary, Visual and Performance Studies at Monash University. She has written extensively in the areas of women's literature, feminism and psychoanalysis.

Nicola Nixon has recently completed her PhD thesis, entitled Contemporary Fantasies of Ancient Hatreds: Ideology and War in former Yugoslavia, in the Department of History and the Ashworth Centre for Social Theory at the University of Melbourne.

Marguerite Nolan is a lecturer in Australian Studies at ACU National. She recently completed her PhD in Indigenous Australian literature at the University of Stirling. She researches and has published in the area of cultural studies in Australia, with particular attention to racialised and gendered identifications and imposture in Australia.

Marjorie O'Loughlin teaches philosophy and social theory in the Faculty of Education at the University of Sydney. She has carried out research into young Australians' conceptions of identity, citizenship and belonging and is further developing this work by means of an ARC Discovery Grant. Her current writing is on the theme of embodiment, 'place' and education.

Robert Reynolds is an Australian Research Council Fellow in the School of Policy and Practice, The University of Sydney. He is the author of *From Camp to Queer: Remaking the Australian Homosexual* (MUP, 2002). He is in training as a psychotherapist.

John Rickard has a longstanding interest in biography and autobiography, and is the author of *H. B. Higgins: The Rebel as Judge* and *A Family Romance: The Deakins at Home*. He is an honorary professorial fellow at Monash University.

Christina Twomey is a Lecturer in the School of Historical Studies at Monash University. She has published in the areas of gender, war and captivity, and is currently writing a book about the internment of Australian women by the Japanese in World War II.

kylie valentine's PhD is from the Department of Gender Studies at the University of Sydney. She is the author of *Psychoanalysis, Psychiatry and Modernist Literature*, published by Palgrave.

Introduction: psychoanalysis, histories and identities

Joy Damousi and Robert Reynolds

PSYCHOANALYSIS, writes Joseph Schwartz, is 'arguably the single most important intellectual development of the twentieth century'.[1] However one judges psychoanalysis as a practice, it is indisputable that its ideas have been historically influential in various forums for understanding interior life and accounting for human action. Over the past thirty years, psychoanalytic concepts have been re-evaluated as several disciplines have appropriated Freudian ideas to interrogate the relationships between culture, the self, identity and the unconscious. The theoretical shifts emerging from poststructuralist and postcolonialist paradigms have inspired a new look at the ways in which psychoanalytic theory can illuminate the intersection between individual and collective identity and society.

The essays in this volume are concerned with exploring the various aspects of the vexed and multifaceted relationship between psychoanalysis and history. In the simplest terms, viewing psychoanalysis and history as professional practices and as bodies of knowledge, this intersection of the two is premised on the belief that the past shapes the present. As psychoanalysis draws on individual memory of past events to unlock the unconscious, and to offer an understanding of how those 'events . . . organise the present', so too has recent historical work insisted that history is defined in the present, subject to rewriting and revision relevant to the preoccupations of the moment.[2] In these endeavours memory is the bridge shared by both psychoanalysis and history, for the processes of remembering and forgetting are central to both practices. Psychoanalysis insists on the need to explore

1

why and how we remember, forget and repress the things we do, whilst history is also concerned with selective memory, revision and the ways in which the narratives of the past are contingent and contested.

Historians have been notoriously resistant to uses of psychoanalytic theory because, it has been argued, figures of the past cannot be psychoanalysed.[3] According to some critics, to adopt such an approach would be to venture into the realm of 'baseless speculation', and pursue a path of 'irrelevance, irresponsibility, and vulgarity'.[4] But, as Christopher Forth points out in his essay in this volume, to utilise some of Sigmund Freud's ideas does not necessitate the application of all aspects of Freudian thought to an analysis of history. As we shall see, there is some historical work which has utilised Freudian concepts to a significant extent, but in large part historians remain ambivalent because the realm of the unconscious cannot be evidenced. Forth's point highlights the way in which those historians who have applied psychoanalytic theory have done so eclectically and selectively.

What have historians found useful in psychoanalytic theory? Perhaps the historian who has attempted the most comprehensive application of such theory is Peter Gay. In his work *Freud for Historians* Gay argues for historians to adopt a more psychoanalytic approach to the past in order to examine the self and the irrational in history with a depth and complexity that is usually lacking in historical accounts of human behaviour. Historians have certainly 'not been unmindful of potent irrationalities in the past', he observes, but when compelled to deal with 'concealed and contradictory emotions', they have done so 'with visible aversion, and have turned away after feeding their readers with a few observations borrowed from commonsense psychology'.[5] Gay for one has tackled such issues directly. In his path-breaking four-volume work on the bourgeois experience, Gay uses Freud's theories on dreams, fantasies, slips of the tongue and linguistic expressions to illuminate the intersections between the self, culture and society. In the latest volume, *The Naked Heart*, Gay explores 'the fascinating spectacle of nineteenth-century bourgeois struggling for inwardness',[6] and examines 'the nineteenth century preoccupation with the self, to the point of neurosis'.[7] Towards this end, Gay draws on Freud's belief that the self was both stable and unstable, in conflict, and shaped by internal as well as external forces. In looking at inner life, Gay argues that better understanding can only be found by examining the deeper 'reaches of the mind' which would be otherwise missed.[8] Freud's theorisations of the ego and superego interacting with cultural forces become the basis from which Gay explores the tensions between the individual's needs and desires, and those of civilisation.[9]

These issues of the intersection between self, society and culture form the basis of the work of others who use psychoanalytic categories to examine past human behaviour. One of the most notable of these studies is

Lyndal Roper's pioneering work, *Oedipus and the Devil*. Roper utilises psycho-analysis to examine individual and collective subjectivity, the irrational, the unconscious and the relationship between the psychic and the physical in the context of witchcraft and early modern Europe. Like Gay, she argues that historians often write 'as if social change impinges directly and uni-formly upon the individual's mental structure, as if the psyche were a kind of blank sheet for social processes to write upon'.[10] In exploring the con-nection between the psyche and the body, Roper draws on insights from the psychoanalyst theorists Melanie Klein and Julia Kristeva to examine the boundaries between self and other. Individual subjectivity can never be understood, she writes, unless there is an understanding of the 'subjectivity of psychology'. Without making the connection between the social and the psychic, Roper asserts, historians cannot adequately conceptualise change, nor will they 'truly encounter the past'.[11]

Feminist historians have also seen some parallels between their work and that of psychoanalysis. Sally Alexander has been at the forefront of such theorisations. Alexander argues that what is central 'to both feminism and psychoanalysis is the discovery of a subjective history through image, symbol and language'. There is, she insists, 'a close proximity between the concept of the unconscious and the unspoken histories of women's lives at the very foundation of psychoanalysis'.[12] For Alexander, the 'psychoanalytic notion of sexual difference in historical work cannot be insisted upon', as to jettison the unconscious, is to 'lose the concept of psychic instability'.[13] Other feminist historians have also adopted this perspective, in more eclec-tic ways. Leonore Davidoff has, for instance, drawn on Freud to investigate the psychic states which underlie various relationships in and outside of the Victorian family.[14]

Another branch of history that has emerged using psychological states as theoretical categories of historical analysis is that of the history of emo-tions. In this field it is the psychological, rather than the psychoanalytic, that frames understanding. Jane Lewis and Peter N. Stearns write that the history of emotions 'coincides with growing interest in emotions in several branches of psychology, philosophy, sociology, and anthropology'.[15] Although some in this field draw on psychoanalysis as well,[16] it is the insights from psycho-logy that inform historical analysis.[17]

Historians have also sought to investigate the theoretical dimensions of the relationship between history and psychoanalysis. Karl Figlio has explored the philosophical relationship between the disciplines of history and psychoanalysis. 'Psychic reality' and 'historical reality' are interrelated, he contends, and cultures as well as individuals 'hold unconscious thera-peutic wishes towards both internal and external worlds'.[18] Michel de Certeau has also focused on similarities between the two, noting how both history and psychoanalysis explore the ways in which the present is shaped in the past through memory.[19] Others such as Daniel Pick have placed Freud's work within broader historical writings. Focusing on the history of the crowd, Pick asks how Freud's paper on group psychology can 'bear upon nationalism and national identity'. He argues that Freud's 'foray into group psychology', 'cannot simply be consigned to the methodological past' as Freud poses problems of a political and psychological nature. Pick reflects on how Freud's work sheds light on the psychological processes of identity formation and how these are also shaped by national identifications, a theme elaborated on in Part III of this book.[20]

In this collection our contributors are similarly preoccupied with issues of the fluid, dynamic and historical relationship between self and society. In the opening essay Catharine Coleborne takes as the focus of her study the historical understanding of 'madness' and points to the ways in which 'the inner worlds and emotional lives of the mad' remain elusive. In histories of psychoanalysis, she argues, the 'mad' are strangely absent; but the history of madness—where the emphasis has been on asylums—is an integral part of psychoanalysis and should be incorporated within in it. Gender is taken as a given in this discussion, as Coleborne alerts us to the central role of femininity in any analysis of formations of identity.

Taking the examination of another type of gendered subjectivity as her starting point—that of masculinity—Joy Damousi shares this concern with the intersection between gender, psychoanalysis and history. In her examination of psychoanalysis in Australia during the interwar years, she explores the different ways in which psychoanalysis was utilised by intellectuals. Situating her argument within debates of the place of interiority within Australian culture, Damousi shows how dream analysis and issues of sexuality in particular were being read and interpreted by those Westerners who looked to Freudian frameworks to make sense of their unconscious world.

A similar but more widespread trend was under way in Britain at this time, as kylie valentine shows in her consideration of interdisciplinarity and literary representations of the self. During the interwar period, 'egoism' and the 'ego' were terms appropriated by those in upper-class British literary circles, in their modern endeavour to define and redefine the self. As valentine shows, these trends were historical: they were closely aligned to developments in psychology and philosophy, and a wider secularisation of society. The other aspect of the self being developed during the interwar years was that of the traumatic potential of memory, where many English writers became, like Freud himself, concerned with the importance of memory and non-linear time in the making of the self.

The chapters in Part I, in various ways, connect psychoanalysis to broader historical phenomena and stress the eclectic nature of psychoanalysis and the ways in which it is shaped by the moment in which it emerges. In his essay on psychoanalysis and homosexuality, Robert Reynolds investigates how psychoanalysis stigmatised homosexuals as perverse subjects for much of the twentieth century. He cites how in the years after his death Freud's liberal analytic approach to homosexuality was whittled away. This was especially marked in the United States during the late 1940s and 1950s, where a Cold War cultural conservatism held sway. In response gay, lesbian and queer activists have been equally dismissive of psychoanalytic knowledge. Reynolds argues that we need to move away from the dichotomies which have constituted these debates, and instead utilise the genuine insights into self-identity offered by such psychoanalytic theorists as Melanie Klein, Donald Winnicott and Heinz Kohut. In arguing for an eclectic and creative deployment of psychoanalysis in relation to homosexuality and gender, Reynolds underlines the need for a recognition of uncertain and contingent identities and sexualities in the new millennium.

In the final piece of Part I, the problematic relationship between Freud and anthropology is thrown into sharp relief. By putting into historical context Freud's theory of the Oedipal moment, Maggie Nolan poses a timely question: how can we discuss the relationship between psychoanalysis and colonialism without considering concepts such as fantasy, desire, projection and displacement? She argues that these issues are at the very heart of the colonial project. It is to the 'disruptive potential' of psychoanalysis that Nolan turns to consider the historical development of anthropology and colonialism. To remove 'the unconscious or psychic motivation from analysis' of colonialism would be misguided. Freud's faith in science should not detract from exploring 'the psychic world of the colonising Western subject', which she argues is fundamentally a historical project which sheds significant light on our understandings of the history of colonialism.

What links these chapters is a consideration of the complex and paradoxical relationship between psychoanalysis and modernity. Taking her cue from Foucault, Coleborne traces what we might call a prehistory, or genealogy, of psychoanalysis. She situates the developmental origins of psychoanalytic theory and practice within the normalising institutions of modernity, most notably the asylum. Coleborne offers an implicit critique of contemporary historians who deploy psychoanalytic concepts. Her concern is understated but nonetheless clear. Psychoanalysis, Coleborne suggests, is heavily implicated in the modern project of governing the soul. As historians uncover and critique this project, psychoanalytic theory should be used cautiously.

Damousi's analysis of how in interwar Australia, when the rational was privileged, it was to the irrational that analytic enthusiasts turned to find the truth of the self, points to a deeper paradox in the relationship between psychoanalysis and modernity. Freud and the early psychoanalysts imagined themselves as the brave prophets of a new, post-traditional world. The myths and illusions of the traditional world were to be relinquished for the scientific findings of psychoanalysis. But by situating the decentred individual at the heart of this modern body of knowledge, psychoanalysis undercut its own certainties. Nothing and nobody was ever fully knowable, for the unconscious would always return to subvert the most ordered of plans and lives. Even analysts were not immune from the caprice of the unconscious, as a growing appreciation of transference and counter-transference in the analytic space revealed. Damousi touches on this in her case study of B. S. Jones's diary of his analysis. Whilst he recorded his dreams in the hope that they would provide a key to his unconscious, Damousi suggests Jones had an audience in mind—his analyst. Thus 'the diarist's sense of self is shaped in an interactive way with his analyst'. Damousi's observation takes us some distance from classical psychoanalysis's modernist imagining of the analyst as a blank screen, the neutral purveyor of scientific insights, towards a more postmodern understanding of psychoanalysis, in which the self is always formed in the contingent space of intersubjectivity.

Some antecedents of postmodernity in Freudian psychoanalysis are also found by valentine. She argues that interdisciplinarity, a concept central to postmodernism, 'is present at the making of psychoanalysis and modernism'. Although no unabashed proponent of psychoanalytic theory—indeed she muses that it may be nearing the limits of its usefulness to critical theory—valentine does note a flaw in contemporary interdisciplinary criticism of psychoanalysis. Such criticism frequently berates psychoanalysis for its claim to universalism and its refusal of situated knowledge; but, as valentine demonstrates, the imperialist reach of psychoanalysis may well be the product of its own interdisciplinary formation. This secret history of interdisciplinarity might give its contemporary enthusiasts some pause, or at least help persuade them that the endeavour of historical inquiry is not yet moribund.

Nolan and Reynolds continue valentine's task of pushing psychoanalysis beyond its modern moorings and into a reflexive critique of its own knowledge and processes. Both deploy psychoanalytic tools even as they critique psychoanalysis's twentieth-century claims to truth. Nolan uses psychoanalysis against itself to reveal the mechanisms of displacement and substitution in Freud's anthropological formulation of the Oedipus complex. Similarly, Reynolds draws on Kleinian theory to illuminate the part-object function homosexuality has played in psychoanalytic theory and practice. This deployment of psychoanalysis against itself is a delicate balancing act, for it is critical and admiring in the same stroke. Ironic, too, in that psychoanalysis has long privileged the toleration of ambivalence.

Questions of identity, the self and the role of the unconscious, in the context of history and psychoanalysis, intersect most explicitly in the genre of biography. This genre, which includes aspects of both the individual and the collective, is the subject of Part II. Judith Brett opens this theme with an overview of the ways in which psychoanalytic ideas—especially those of Kohut, Freud and Klein—can be utilised in writing political biography. Using her own study of Robert Menzies as an example, Brett shows how Heinz Kohut's psychology of the self, with its emphasis upon ambitions and ideals, can be utilised to speculate on the inner world and public motivations of political figures. From Klein, Brett borrows the key concepts of projection and introjection as a means of understanding 'the traffic between the inner and the outer world'.

More generally, Brett challenges a number of myths in relation to the genre of psychoanalytic biography and attempts to debunk these in her discussion. These include a focus exclusively on sexuality and the belief that analysing individuals involves examining the workings of 'ahistorical drives'. On the contrary, the advantage of psychoanalysis, Brett argues, is that it 'provides the biographer with a grammar of the emotions to guide [the] interpretative task' of analysing their subjects' emotions. To do otherwise is to rely only on 'common sense, religion and literature' and therefore to ignore 'patterns not otherwise discernible'. The relationship between the public and the private is central to this discussion. Brett highlights the point —common to the pieces in this section—that psychobiography is founded on the history of private life and the psychoanalytic ways in which this impinges on the public persona.

John Rickard takes up this challenge of the public, the private and the historical in his examination of the dynamics of the Victorian family. Rickard attempts such reading in this consideration of Alfred Deakin and Henry Higgins and the ways in which family relationships play out their particular emotional lives. In doing so, Rickard challenges our understanding of the Victorian middle-class family, often regarded as 'hidebound and morally censorious'. As he shows, the families of neither Higgins nor Deakin fit this model, for 'within the bounds of the topics which could be addressed (particularly by women) emotion could be given full reign; indeed the culture often encouraged the fervent expression of such emotion'. In this middle-class Victorian context, Rickard observes that it was often language which was the 'bearer of emotion'.

By writing himself into his histories of Deakin and Higgins, Rickard allows us further insight into the way inner and outer worlds intersect, both for the historian's subjects and the historian himself. Rickard relates how his twice-weekly therapy in Los Angeles with Victor, who was 'pretty much a conventional Freudian' analyst, and the concomitant reflection on his own childhood moulded his reading of Deakin and Higgins's familial lives. As Rickard's chapter unfolds, this influence of Freudian psychoanalysis becomes clear. Almost with an analyst's ear, Rickard is drawn to the free-associative elements of Deakin's and Higgins's writing, in which he finds examples of repetition, displacement, metaphor, distortion, neurotic conflict, sibling rivalry, guilt and reparation. This is the grand and tragic material of Freudian analysis, with its emphasis on drives and defences. And while there are legitimate critiques that such a metapsychology can slide towards the ahistorical, Rickard makes a compelling historical case for the use of Freudian theory in the study of Victorian families.

The influence of the familial on public lives and the historian's use of language to discern this dynamic are also central to Bain Attwood's biographical study of anthropologist Donald Thomson. Attwood argues that Thomson's 'emotionally powerful identification' with the plight of Indigenous Australians originated from the earlier traumas of his childhood and reflected his own 'worse childhood fears of abandonment or exile'. Through a careful examination of Thomson's language and the conflation of his identity with that of Indigenous Australians, Attwood explores the psychology and politics of empathy. The key psychological concepts Attwood deploys in tracing Thomson's passionate commitment to the cause of Aboriginal rights are idealisation, projection and identification. It is important to note that in explaining Thomson's political ideals through these terms and via his childhood, Attwood in no way diminishes the significance and courage of Thomson's activism, or the importance of history.

Both Rickard and Attwood situate their case studies firmly within a historical context and connect the psychology of their protagonists to that context. In the case of the former it is the middle-class Victorian family; in the latter, the dynamics of colonialism and race relations. The personal histories which inform their discussions provide another layer of interconnectedness between the psychoanalytic dimensions of the relationship between public and private life.

In concluding this section on biography, Christopher Forth takes us from a concern with the self to a more recent intellectual fascination with the body. The leading voice in a 'history of bodies' has been Michel Foucault, and while Forth happily acknowledges the value in mapping the discourses that constitute the modern body, he ponders the limits of social constructionist thought. Forth asks: is the idea of interiority simply a colonisation of the inside by the exterior? He suspects not, positing instead a dynamic relationship between inner and outer as lived and experienced through the body. Psychoanalysis has had much to say about how the body experiences the inner and outer as one, not least through introjection and projection. Reading the nineteenth-century journals of French philosopher Henri-Frédéric Amiel, Forth thus turns to Freudian and post-Freudian thought to elaborate on how 'physical integrity could be so emotionally invested as to become virtually synonymous with selfhood'. In considering such issues, Forth contextualises the histories of hygiene, medicine and morality, and their relationship to 'normative modes of masculine identity'. Finally, in bringing theories of the embodied unconscious and abjection to bear upon a history of bodies, Forth deploys psychoanalysis lightly, as 'one interpretative tool among many'.

Moving from individual histories to the exploration of group experiences has always posed a challenge for psychoanalysis, as John Cash notes in the concluding chapter of this book. Biography can at least approximate, vicariously, the theories of the consulting room, whether through the analysis of texts or interviews. The best practitioners of this art—and here Judith Brett and the late Graham Little spring to mind—address 'the contingent effects of social process (and specific, often traumatic, events), by analysing the ways in which such processes and events mark themselves upon the subject'. Matters become more complicated the further one moves away from the study of an individual or a specific grouping with a common and shared identity. At this point, suggests Cash, there must be some attempt to more systematically theorise social processes. Nowhere is this more pertinent than in the analysis of nationalism and national identities, the subject of Part III.

Miriam Dixson opens this section by focusing on the example of Anglo-Australian identity. She charts the link between nationalism, identity and the social imaginary, which encompasses institutions, language and history. Drawing on the theories of Cornelius Castoriadis, Dixson explicates the way in which the 'imaginary institution of society' and those institutions that shape 'imaginary significations' such as language, laws, customs, techniques, arts, topography and climate can be applied to understanding the Australian imaginary. To this list she adds the 'experience of convictism, the originary power of an authoritarian, centralised state, Anglo-Irish rancour, and race and sex relations'. It is within this discussion that Dixson argues that early Anglo qualities have been sustained over Australia's history. These qualities, Dixson suggests, have been crucial to Australia's particular experience of 'the project of autonomy', and remain so today, despite the vibrant overlay of non-Anglo cultures. Dixson's position, detailed in her 1999 book, *The Imaginary Australian*, has not been without its critics, and in this chapter she responds by elaborating on her 30-year intellectual journey through psychoanalytic theory. Historians generally have not greatly taken to psychoanalysis in Australia, and Dixson's willingness to deploy diverse strands of psychoanalytic thought—from Erik Erikson through to Melanie Klein and, more recently, the philosopher-analyst Cornelius Castoriadis—has been impressively, and presciently, eclectic.

Kleinian thought and object relations theory more widely appear in Marjorie O'Loughlin's analysis of the ties that bind individuals to a sense of nationhood. In studying the sources of national attachment, O'Loughlin argues that the significance of place has been overlooked. While not denying the importance of an ethnic or civic core in debates about national attachment, O'Loughlin draws on Klein, Winnicott, and Kohut's self psychology, as well as a European philosophical tradition, to suggest that a sense of national belonging is 'interwoven with attachment, with a sense of being in-place'. O'Loughlin uses Klein to demonstrate how fantasy infuses national imaginings, in ways that are both potentially creative and destructive, and Winnicott and Kohut to further detail the social, shared nature of fantasy. The broader cultural significance of these theories, she argues, is that they can be used to study 'such phenomena as attachment to the nation, national feeling and identity'. She does this here with a phenomenological appreciation of place, or more specifically, the ways in which embodied individuals experience history 'in place'. Both approaches (the psychoanalytic and the phenomenological) may be particularly useful in studying contemporary discourses of national attachment in Australia. The 2001 Federal election, for example, saw the skilful political manipulation of fantasies of national belonging and security in ways that were chillingly successful. Psychoanalysis and an appreciation of place and history can help decode these political messages, although the task of rebutting their power and appeal may well be more onerous.

Nicola Nixon returns to the theme of particular enduring national discourses in her paper on the imaginary in the Balkan region. Nixon expands on this topic in the context of the war in the Balkans, where she frames the repetition of the discourse of ancient Balkan animosities in terms of social fantasy. Nixon links fantasy—'operating in unconscious, habitual social practices rather than cognitive thought'—to the social linkage of imagined communities. In ideological terms, fantasy structures 'unconscious desire' and impacts on social processes beyond their immediate expression in discourse. Through this prism, Nixon explores the fantasy of Balkan tribalism —termed the 'ancient hatreds thesis'—which, she argues, structured the very mechanisms of the international peace process, and constructed and legitimated the violent destruction in Yugoslavia. Her chapter, which charts the relationship between the imaginary, the material and the discursive in one corner of world politics, gives weight to Dennis Altman's call for a psychoanalytic materialist study of international relations.[21] In all three chapters in this section, the various forms of nationalism and their psycho-analytic expression are firmly grounded within, and gain meaning from, the historical context which has shaped their very expression.

The theme of trauma and memory has in recent times been developed and articulated by scholars using psychoanalytic frameworks to reinterpret historical events. In memories of war, the place of traumatic subjectivity has become central to historical analysis.[22] This theme is at the centre of the essays by Esther Faye and Christina Twomey. What Faye describes as the 'therapeutic use of history' informs her study of second-generation Holocaust survivors. Using a Lacanian framework, she examines the relationship between trauma, *jouissance* and history in two ways. First, she questions the recent efforts by some commentators for a recognition of a shared past between Jews and Germans. Second, through an examination of the writing of the Jewish-Australian writer Yvonne Fein, she asks whether children of Holocaust survivors can detach themselves from a 'masochistic enjoyment of it' and 'stage' history instead. In this paper, a Lacanian psychoanalytic understanding of history sheds light on the complex Jewish–German relationship; on the second generation of Holocaust survivors; and on the contested nature of Jewish identity itself. In another consideration of the traumas of war, Twomey takes the experiences of civilian internees during World War II as the subject of her inquiry. One of the key themes to emerge from this study is that trauma is not experienced in a homogenous way. Women especially drew on particular discourses over time to express the legacy of their traumas, reflecting the historical specificity of how people experience, relate and understand trauma. The relationship between trauma, psychoanalytic theory and historical narrative is drawn together in this discussion as the point is made, following Cathy Caruth, that the trau-matised 'carry an impossible history within them'.[23]

The relationship between psychoanalysis and trauma has been the focus of many studies—especially those analysing war and the Holocaust. The origins of psychoanalysis, as Adam Phillips has observed, are immersed in war, for it was 'partly made out of materials of war, its casualties and its language'.[24] Faye and Twomey draw on the uses for history of this relation-ship. In Twomey's account, it is the 'unexpressed history' which is exam-ined in the process of that traumatic history becoming absorbed into the present rather than *returning* as an 'alternative reality'. Faye spotlights the ways in which the taming of the relationship between German and Jew promotes a certain type of history that moves beyond a 'deadly fascination' with the Holocaust. In each of these pieces, our understanding of the cul-ture of the historical period—the nineteenth century, the interwar years and the present—is illuminated and extended by and examination of psycho-analysis either as a historical phenomena or as an explanatory tool.

Finally, the texts and archives which are used to explore these themes add a further richness to our understandings of how the various and complex intersections between psychoanalysis and history are produced. The case history is examined by Coleborne as a particular source where subjectivities are interpreted and defined. Patient casebooks are themselves 'histories', she argues. Diaries have long been identified as precious and illuminating texts which can expose the conscious and unconscious thoughts of those living and dead. Coleborne draws on a diary to enter into the emotional space of her protagonist. In her examination of another type of diary—one documenting dreams—Damousi examines the formation of masculinity through self-analysis.

Both valentine and Faye draw on a different kind of text—literature— to explore the ways in which these can also provide productive means of reading the workings of the self, ego and the unconscious. In particular valentine points to the narratives and various institutions which promoted ideas of psychoanalysis; these were no more revealing than in the work of literary doyens of the modern period, such as James Joyce, Virginia Woolf and H. D. Faye examines the crime detective novel, *April Fool*, to examine how such a text lends itself to a complex psychoanalytic reading like the one offered here. In drawing also on the confessional, Faye shares with Twomey an interest in this narrative form as a means of exploring trauma and psychoanalysis. The confessional mode, which in many respects is evident in all of the sources used in Part I, also points to the intersection between the private and the public and to the ways in which issues of the 'private' become political.

The relationship between literature and psychoanalysis has aroused far less resistance among literary critics than historians, as those working in the fields of literary studies and cultural studies have often championed the uses of psychoanalysis in exploring interiority and the unconscious through textual analysis.[25] Both share an interest in language, and 'an investigation of character', while the intersection of psychoanalysis and literature with history is often to be found in exploration of time and memory.[26] Rose Lucas takes us through the relationship between the literary form and psychoanalysis, where it is the 'telling of stories' that offers a 'pathway to comprehension and redemption from the oppressive power of what is hidden or repressed'. Through an examination of Margaret Atwood's *Alias Grace* Lucas highlights the central role of narrative in both literature and psychoanalysis and how in both mediums it becomes almost impossible to know and define the elusive concept of subjectivity. Both in being an examination of the history of psychoanalysis itself, and in using such narrative frameworks to tease the reader, Atwood's novel, as Lucas points out, 'reaffirms our desire to know and define the concept of subjectivity almost despite the impossibility of doing so'.

In the closing chapter of this volume, John Cash also touches on the frequent and significant role trauma plays in the constitution of the subject. The subject, he argues, extending psychoanalytic theory, is doubly decentred —first through the dynamic unconscious and then through the rules of the field of ideology. He contends that it is as a doubly decentred subject 'that we find our place and take our place in the ongoing history of the present'. From here, Cash takes us on a tour of social theory's attempt to grapple with this double decentring. Cash critiques the ways in which social theory has appropriated psychoanalysis as a theory of socialisation, thereby flattening out a conceptualisation of the subject. What is lost in this melancholic transfer is what Cash details as the very stuff of history: 'the conflicted, contested, dynamic making and remaking of identity and social relations in the contingent here and now'. In his closing paragraphs, appropriately enough, Cash returns to Freud for inspiration in sketching out an approach to history and the unconscious that does not stumble at the social.

The aim of this collection is to highlight the eclectic and diverse application of aspects of psychoanalytic thought within concepts of history and the past which include issues relating to both the individual and the collective. In utilising a broad range of approaches, concepts, categories and frameworks, these essays point to the rich and varied terrain of what is termed the 'psychoanalytic' and to how these can be connected to, and shaped by, historical considerations. American historian and psychoanalytic theorist Fred Weinstein has recently noted that the history of psychoanalysis —and its likely future—is one of fragmentation. In this volume alone, our contributors have drawn upon the work of Freud, Klein, Kohut, Winnicott, Erickson, Jacques Lacan, Castoriadis and Slavoj Zizek in their psychoanalytic readings of history. Each of these psychoanalytic theorists differs in their conceptualisation of the subject in history, and their use, accordingly, produces different histories of the present.

As Reynolds notes in his chapter, psychoanalysis in the twenty-first century is a very broad church, and its congregation fractious. A historian using classical Freudian theory might choose to study the operation of drives and defences in any one historical moment. A Kleinian might look at the splitting, projection and projective identification of innate aggressive fantasies, and the acts of reparation that could follow from such phantasmic processes. Conversely, a Winnicottian might pay greater attention to environmental factors and to how inner and outer worlds meet in transitional objects and phenomena. The follower of Kohut could privilege a history of the self, and the various transferential experiences—mirroring, idealisation and twinship—that constitute this self. Using the ego psychological-inspired work of Eric Erikson, a historian might discern the building blocks and stages of identity, not simply in the life of an individual, but also the collective and the nation. From the writing of Lacan, Zizek and Castoriadis, the historian can bring complex theories of the imaginary to bear upon a history of social formations.

All of these approaches are deployed, in varying and eclectic degrees, in the essays that follow. In writing histories that pay due attention to the canny and the uncanny, this eclecticism is welcome. Such a diverse application of psychoanalytic theory is also perfectly within the tradition of psychoanalysis; for, as Weinstein observes, 'far from being the authoritatively controlled and easily managed discipline that critics have often claimed it to be, psychoanalysis is and always has been anarchic in its tendencies, resembling too much its clinical subject, the idiosyncratic subject'. In this volume psychoanalytic connections are further mediated by class, race, ethnicity, sexuality and gender, themselves historical categories which have often been discussed outside of understandings of the rational, the logical and common sense. By drawing attention to the emotional aspects of the relationships and identities which are shaped along these axes, this volume coheres around the notion that emotional life has a history that is contested in the cracks and fault lines between the past and the present. In the writing of these idiosyncratic histories, psychoanalysis remains a valuably uncanny companion.

I

Analysing modernity

1

Hearing the 'speech of the excluded': re-examining 'madness' in history

Catharine Coleborne

I N 1984 SALLY ALEXANDER suggested that the topic of subjectivity was an inescapable part of writing history in her influential essay, 'Women, Class and Sexual Difference in the 1830s and '40s'.[1] Alexander's immediate primary audience for this essay, an international community of feminist historians, was excited by the apparent trend towards examining the 'inner worlds' of women in the past. While not the first to bring psychoanalytic praxis 'into history', Alexander's work is now furthered by historians who have been convinced by her claim that the 'unconscious and phantasy' are 'working like alchemy among us'.[2] Her work provides me with a useful starting point for this chapter as I consider another, different problem for historians. Alexander's subjects were working women and political women. They were not incarcerated inside nineteenth- or early twentieth-century institutions. For Alexander, these women's subjectivities were incomplete, as subjectivity is always fractured and partial. However, the problem of 'madness' in the past poses different questions. Despite sharing the characteristics of all subjectivities and (self-)representations, the subjectivities of 'mad' women and men are more difficult to access. Their voices are more often represented by others, and moreover the scholarly histories of these representations often shut down the possibility of our engagement with their words, their agency, and with them.

The history of 'madness' before the twentieth century has generally been constituted in ways that limit our access to the inner worlds or emotional lives of the 'mad'. This very broad field makes a number of forays into

17

the realm of discursive approaches from current psychiatric medicine which, at critical junctures, sometimes fail to understand madness in the past. One such discursive detour is a practice known as making a 'retrospective diagnosis', or assigning a 'late twentieth-century [psychiatric] label' to 'symptoms recorded in the case notes of the past'. This is a practice largely conducted by psychiatrists writing history.[3] Thus the worlds of the mad have been invisible within histories of 'selfhood', subjectivity and the development of psychoanalysis. Some histories, including edited collections of the writings of women and men incarcerated in the nineteenth century, have appeared in the past decade.[4] Most scholarship has focused on the asylum, committals to it, and the medical and social worlds within the asylum's walls.

This chapter draws on extant patient case histories from the first psychiatric institutions in the colony of Victoria, Australia. The Yarra Bend Asylum was established in 1848, and another metropolitan asylum was built at Kew in 1871. Their populations grew rapidly throughout the nineteenth century and raised the spectre of madness as a colonial contagion. Recent histories, including my own work, have used patient casebooks but have shown patients' lives and experiences to be highly circumscribed and mediated through these texts, or they have used them to create asylum population profiles. Yet asylum patient case histories have an important place in helping us to recover the subjectivities of the mad.[5] This chapter illustrates that, from the fragments in patient casebooks from asylums and unpublished personal accounts of madness, historians are able to access the emotional lives of the mad in the past. It does this by re-examining two sources from the history of madness in nineteenth-century colonial Australia: Catherine Currie's (self-)representation of what she called her 'distraction' in the 1880s, produced *outside* the asylum; and the patient casebook history constructed around her experience inside the asylum.[6]

Genealogies: histories of 'madness' and 'psychiatry'

In the last decade, a small amount of scholarship in this large field has usefully linked the histories of 'psychiatry' and 'psychological' practices—incorporating ideas about psychoanalysis and psychotherapy—to histories of the nineteenth-century asylum and its techniques. In general, despite the suggestive work in the 1960s and 1970s by Michel Foucault, there has been a tendency to separate these scholarly areas. The histories of madness and the asylum, and those of psychoanalysis, have *not* traced continuities, but rather have seen themselves as quite separate projects.[7] Yet, as more than one commentator has noted, Foucault saw psychoanalysis as the virtual 'fulfilment' of the aims of the asylum, and he provided historians with a context 'for writing the history of psychoanalysis' by situating psychoanalytic theory and praxis within the context of 'normalizing' institutions.[8]

Making this leap here might seem to be an implicit critique of the psychoanalytic project for historians like Alexander. This chapter argues that by retrieving aspects of Foucault's understanding of the way madness in the past can be read and understood through its representations, historians might see the possibilities in Foucault's reading of the history of psychiatry. It is also important to acknowledge that Foucault meant to produce 'histories of the present'. If we are to fully appreciate the psychoanalytic turn in history writing about psychological practices, it is useful to deploy Foucault's concept of the 'archaeology of knowledge', as an 'archaeological investigation or "history of the present" views the conditions of possibility of knowledge as central to the project of understanding the constitution of contemporary psychological objects'.[9] Thus the history of madness in the asylum should not be viewed as separate from, or as a historical backdrop to, the project of psychoanalytic history, but should appear as an integral part of it.

The asylum's 'everyday practices' in inscribing identities led to the creation of certain 'psychological vocabularies'.[10] As historians have argued more recently, early twentieth-century practices around psychoanalysis, within a popular psychiatric framework, came to have cultural authority because of the established authority of the techniques of the asylum.[11] This cultural authority was gained by psychiatrists because of the techniques they developed and not because the institution itself had authority, although the two are related.[12] Foucault went further than this, and saw 'our contemporary world of madness' as inseparable from the discipline of psychiatry and a new 'psychiatric epistemology'. He argued that it was only when inside the asylum—a particular interpretative domain—that madness or 'tragic, wild, scandalous, distressing, incomprehensible acts' became visible.[13] This claim, while it is a useful tool for understanding the history of the asylum, is perhaps too limiting for historians of madness. The world outside the asylum was also an interpretative domain and the asylum's inextricable relationship to this world cannot not be denied. Catherine Currie's diary indicates that outside the asylum in the nineteenth century men and women made evaluations of their own and others' behaviours. When Catherine was considered to be 'ill' her husband, neighbours and friends decided to seek medical advice about her condition. They also made assessments of her mental health based on their understandings of the 'symptoms' of madness.

In 1883 the *Age* newspaper reported two cases of insanity in rural Victoria: one was a case of 'religious mania' and the other a case of the suicide of a young woman. The case of 'religious mania' caused 'great excitement' at Ironbark near Sandhurst when a young man named Henry Keast was 'greatly affected' by the sermon at the United Methodist Church. Henry was 'returned to his home, but did not return to his senses till long afterwards'. His utterances were treated as evidence of 'mania', as the report's title indicated. Henry 'declared that he had been conducted by an angel through Heaven and Hell, in both of which places he had met several acquaintances'. A few days earlier, at Burnt Creek near Horsham, 19-year-old Dora Peeck committed suicide. At the inquiry into her death witnesses attested to the fact that Dora had been ill with severe headaches since her bout of scarlet fever three years before. Witnesses commented on the woman's constant anguish and on her utterance of the phrase, 'I believe I shall go mad: I wish I was dead'. The inquiry found that Dora had drowned herself 'whilst laboring under a fit of insanity'.[14] The utterances of those believed to be mad outside the asylum walls are important because they provide glimpses of madness so often concealed in histories of psychiatry.

Catherine Currie, from Gippsland in Victoria, was also diagnosed as suffering from 'acute mania' in the 1880s. Like Henry Keast she conjured images of hell in her despair, and like Dora Peeck anguish drove her into 'madness'. She felt 'punished' for the accidental death by drowning of her youngest child. Catherine was admitted to the Yarra Bend Asylum by her husband, John, in September 1881 after the death. In her diary she told of her grief; and after her admission to the asylum, her distressed husband wrote about his impressions of the asylum and her confinement.

Patient casebooks provide evidence that family and friends sometimes offered details about the behaviour and symptoms of those they admitted, which were recorded and became part of medical narrative. Margaret Maria M., aged 28, was taken to the metropolitan asylum at Kew by her father in 1874. It was his suggestion that she had first exhibited signs of 'mania'— though this diagnosis was probably made by the asylum—two years before this attack because of 'disappointment in intended marriage'.[15] Another father took his 21-year-old daughter, Helen W., to Yarra Bend suffering from 'Hysterical Mania' due to 'love affairs'.[16] Women were also admitted by their mothers, their nieces and female friends. Those people close to the alleged 'lunatic' noted things like physical appearance, obvious excitement and violent behaviour, together with eccentric and self-destructive acts, as in the case of Charlotte G.'s husband, who advised that his wife had tried to poison herself twice and had 'on one occasion . . . swallowed a dish of kerosene oil'.[17] Such detail was incorporated into published cases in medical journals, where the 'case' was established within medical practice.[18]

Before Freud, the psychiatric 'case' was defined by physicians as a 'history'. The information about inmates in the casebook, or case history, became increasingly detailed in asylums around the western world as the nineteenth century drew to a close. In the early part of the nineteenth century Philippe Pinel and other alienists in France were interested in this method of observing and interviewing patients and composing detailed case histories. By the end of the nineteenth century the style of the casebook was evidence of the 'psychologic method'.[19] In America the casebook was evidence of the impact of the rise in interest in psychopathology. In colonial asylums the casebook mimicked these styles and also became a site for the construction of colonial medical knowledge.[20]

The Yarra Bend casebook captured Catherine for a time in its framework.[21] The entry for 17 September 1881 tells us certain facts about (Anne) Catherine Currie. The book indicated that she was thirty years old, her religion was Church of England, she worked at 'Household duties' and was suffering from 'Acute Mania' and had been for seven or eight weeks prior to admission. The cause of her illness was stated as 'Death of child by drowning'. Catherine's only bodily illness was described: 'Hands and wrists swolen [*sic*] from tying'. The casebook notes were brief and to the point: 'This woman is strong and robust in person and appears healthy. She suffers from acute mania and is very violent and dangerous. She refuses her food and is in all respects difficult to manage'. While this is a description typical of casebook entries, Catherine's 'violence' and sleeplessness had been apparent before her committal.[22]

Like other women in asylums she resisted control. While there was little written about her behaviour for the remainder of her stay at Yarra Bend, it might be assumed that she began to accept controls rather than continue to resist them. This led to her being described as 'much improved', although this was not always the case, as John discovered when he visited her.[23] By 14 October 1881 Catherine was described as 'much improved and . . . now fairly well'. At the end of December she was allowed home on trial under the care of her husband.[24] According to the casebook, Catherine was not formally discharged until October 1883, and she appears to have remained at home after her 'trial' release. Her status as an asylum inmate is unclear in the two years or so in between. In her diaries she told of her painful experience of anxiety and loss in her own words, something which the casebook from Yarra Bend Asylum omitted and was not designed to include. Her husband John also wrote about the experience of committing his wife to an asylum, and the diary reveals a husband's emotional distress at the events surrounding his wife's great grief.

The emphasis on psychotherapy in the twentieth century has possibly diminished the significance of the case history. Mark Micale suggests that aspects of the professional past of psychiatry have been obscured: as he notes, in the late nineteenth century the 'science of the mind' was 'rich and diversified'.[25] In different national contexts, 'mainstream' psychiatry only 'warmed' to psychoanalysis in the 1920s, and prior to this, the different 'disciplines' had independent trajectories.[26] But words and ideas later associated with psychoanalysis were being explored inside asylums: as American historian John C. Burnham has noted, there were American precursors to Freud, and concepts like the unconscious and the 'sexual factors associated with the etiology of hysteria' were in limited circulation, explaining perhaps the later acceptance of Freudian arguments in that context.[27] Philip Cushman also offers what he calls 'a historically situated interpretation' of the rise of the psychoanalytic practice of psychotherapy in the United States, arguing that it was a congruence of factors, including the rise of notions of 'the self' and 'the therapeutic' underlined by the mental hygiene movement, that made the reception of Freud's ideas in that context possible.[28] Historians of British psychiatry also claim a strong link between psychiatry and psychoanalysis.[29] Freud himself attempted to persuade his audience of the relationship between psychiatry and psychoanalysis in his series of lectures on 'Psychoanalysis and Psychiatry'.[30] In Australia following World War I the practice of psychotherapy became more acceptable to psychiatrists, despite conflict over specific issues.[31] But as the following section of this chapter argues, it was both inside and outside the asylum that personal histories became important to individuals suffering episodes of madness.

'Oh had she only talked her troubles over they would have been nothing': Catherine Currie's diary

Catherine's diary description of the death of her youngest child came three weeks after the event occurred. She stopped writing in her diary for this time, and when she resumed the first words she wrote belied the extent of her grief. Then a full description of the death by drowning followed. A part of this much longer account is reproduced below:

> I was getting the Dinner Tea ready, I carried her to the hole to dip a bucket of water. I stood her down and dipped it and she had a drink out the bucket . . . The first thing I saw was a little foam on the water. My heart told me what that was. Oh shall I ever forget it. I looked under the sticks and saw my wee Pet, but oh dear I never though[t] I was too late, as she was such a short time in . . . My heart is breaking and I feel frightened to grieve . . . for fear I am Punished even more severely. for it must have been as a punishment that she was taken from

me like that. I can't help blaming myself for letting her out of my mind . . . [at the burial] I was newly distracted and hardly knew what I was doing, if I do yet. She seems never to be out of my mind . . .[32]

This event was devastating for Catherine. Her words for the anxiety she felt were strong: 'shall I ever forget it'. She was fearful of her grief, felt that the death was a punishment of some kind, and described her state after this experience as being one of 'distraction'. She wrote too of her 'mind', this new site of her worry, anxiety and fear.

The isolation and difficulty of rural life highlighted this emotion of fear. Catherine had been struggling anyway with the pressures of farm life. Before the terrible incident when her youngest child drowned, she expressed some of her fears about bushfires: 'Oh, I am so frightened, fairly miserable—we will have to try and get away from here after this'.[33] The difficulties of supervising and caring for young children were great. She also expressed her frustration when she went to vaccinate her baby on 12 April that year and the doctor did not arrive to perform the inoculation. On 2 September 1881 Catherine recorded reading the news about 'a terrible railway accident' in the newspaper, and an impression of gloom pervades these pages and subsequent diary entries that month. Catherine then had a humiliating experience when she was not able to cash a cheque in town.[34]

The last entry Catherine was able to write in her diary before she was too ill to continue appeared on 8 September 1881. Before he took his wife to Yarra Bend, John began to write in the diary, an act of respect for her own practice of diary keeping, and possibly some solace at the time. But he was also entering the site of her mind, or at least records of some of its more sensible contents. His own mind was preoccupied. He described the process of realising that Catherine needed some kind of professional medical help, the assistance of friends, and wrote of their journey to Melbourne. When he arrived home from the harrowing journey John wrote, 'Come home "home is it". what a change' and there begins his sad record of the emotions around his wife's committal.[35]

John evidently thought little of the asylum when he visited: 'what an establishment'. His first visit to his wife was controlled, and he found it difficult to talk to her: 'they gave me the hint to go away'. This and subsequent visits to Yarra Bend reinforced his sense that Catherine's committal was a 'terrible calamity',[36] and he began to feel dreadfully responsible for her state, wishing she had trusted him to talk to him more and that he had made himself more available for her.[37] Reading her diary gave him an insight into her mind, but the act of entering this private space made him feel responsible for all her feelings. By mid-October his anxiety had increased: 'I have been reading [the diary] & find that I have been to blame in my treatment of my wife I should have known better . . .' He wanted to repair the damage but was still wary, as 'it is near the anniversary of the child's death and I am frightened for that time . . . we made a mistake in not talking it over quickly'.[38] By 29 December 1881 John had mustered the ability to free his wife from Yarra Bend. He had received advice from the doctor who told him the procedure must be formalised, and he marked the day in the diary with two large crosses.

When she returned home and was able to write in the diary again, Catherine said little about her experience of the asylum. But small comments revealed her distaste for its methods of 'healing': 'I have felt so well all day, I think a good rest and sleep is the best Medicine'.[39] Other allusions to her health during that first month include '. . . I feel first rate only weak . . . this is the first day I have written the Book and I have filled in the items from Monday' (13 January) and '. . . I feel first rate and I feel very thankful to my heavenly Father that I am so well' (19 January). Catherine's comments about the role of writing 'the Book' in her recovery and John's remarks about Catherine's experience are significant. They both allude to the importance of 'talking'. He writes, 'Oh had she only talked her troubles over they would have been nothing.' Going over his part in her unhappiness, he laments: 'she almost killed herself. I think she should have known me better but I behaved badly to her a man that is to [*sic*] proud to let a wife know how he loves her will get punished.'[40]

Conclusion

If our contemporary world of madness was born in the asylum, as Foucault asserted, the experiences of those confined within asylums and their attempts to talk and be listened to are a key to understanding the later reception of psychoanalytic practices. Catherine and John insisted on the value of talk, in hesitant ways, and the asylum case recorded her 'noise'. This asylum was not yet ready to admit to the importance of talk, as John could see. But the asylum's 'elliptical' thinking and representations of madness in case notes inscribed the idea of making personal histories from fragments of everyday loss and recovery. For asylum inmates, and for the asylum itself, the case was a 'heuristic fiction that was at the same time real'.[41]

Seeing the historical relationship between psychiatric practices and psychoanalytic practices is immediately convincing to me as a historian of the asylum and its techniques. Historians of the asylum and its nineteenth-century patient populations have based their inquiries on patient casebooks, records that became 'the stuff of [psychiatric] science'. It was here in these records that psychiatrists 'fashioned categories' to address the elusiveness of knowledge about mental breakdown, while at the same time they fashioned psychiatric knowledge itself.[42]

The patient casebook is one text we might use to access stories of madness in the past. Given the paucity of other kinds of accounts of mental breakdown the casebook is in many instances the only text available for this purpose. 'Nothing will remain in the hands of cultural historians', suggested Foucault, 'except the codified methods of confinement, the techniques of medicine, and, on the other hand, the sudden, irruptive inclusion in our language of the speech of the excluded'.[43] Foucault argued that one of the ways 'we' recognise past 'madness' is by seeing it through the evidence of those knowledges that disciplined it. Patient casebooks in the nineteenth century constituted 'techniques', and they also sometimes revealed this 'speech of the excluded', such as the remark recorded about one female patient, Elizabeth W., in 1869: 'she says she is sure she will get well here'.[44] However, where possible, historians might look at the suggestive discursive differences between textual representations of madness, as the sources used here illustrate. Catherine Currie was not sure she would 'get well' in the asylum, unlike Elizabeth and other women who learned to perform their wellness. She wrote in her diary after many years of struggle to be and to appear well: 'I have been unhappy all my life', and later, 'if John had never taken me to a *Mad House* I would have been happy in my children'.[45]

There is an important dialogue between the asylum's case history and Catherine's diary. When historians have attempted to talk about 'what mad people meant to say, what was on their minds', they have often found it difficult to present the mind of the sufferer unmediated by its historical context.[46] The dominant discursive modes of the day cut across attempts to see inside the minds of the mad. Historians have almost unwittingly rendered the period of the asylum as the period in which mad people were silent, with a few exceptions. Catherine Currie was not silent: she used physical means of expression, and she used the idea of writing, or silent 'talk', to be heard.

2

A history of dreams: modernity, masculinity and inner life, 1920s and 1930s

Joy Damousi

In March 1938 the Reverend J. Leighton-Edwell wrote to his friend and colleague Ernest Burgmann, the Anglican Bishop of Goulburn and Canberra, with a request for assistance. He told Burgmann he was trying to

> help a family where the husband is a big problem to the wife and children through some mental derangements apparently resulting from the war. He has weird hallucinations at night of the enemy attacking his house and co. and always has a great jealousy with regard to his wife & her contact with almost *anyone*—male or female, and at times orders and threatens her to stay home for weeks on end.

In his own mind, Leighton-Edwell knew what needed to be done to handle aggressive behaviour and repair psychological damage. 'No doubt', he confidently asserted, 'he should be psycho-analysed, but how to persuade him in that direction is the problem'. He asked Burgmann if he knew the name of an expert, although his perception of how such an expert might go about improving the mind of the inflicted would have horrified even the most liberal of analysts. 'Do you know of an analist [*sic*]', he asked, 'who would perhaps call at the home where the man would stay & try to do the job, as a more or less casual visitor? I can think of no other possible solution. Any help you can suggest would be appreciated greatly.'[1] This was not the only request Burgmann had received for such a recommendation. A Miss Frost wrote to him in May 1939, with a far weightier qualification for the sort of analyst she required than a preparedness to make a home visit. Frost wrote

26

that she would 'be most grateful' if Burgmann could recommend 'a clever psycho-analyst in Sydney'.[2]

While the influence of psychoanalysis in intellectual circles and within the medical profession has been the subject of several short studies in Australia, cultural historians have in large part neglected the writing of psychoanalysis in its own right.[3] Towards correcting this absence I first consider some of the eclectic uses to which psychoanalytic ideas were put during the interwar years in Australia to contextualise discussions about psychoanalysis and the unconscious. The left-wing priest Ernest Burgmann, the medical doctor Roy Coupland Winn and the eugenicist and feminist Marion Piddington represented three distinctive responses to Freudian ideas about the unconscious. For Burgmann it was a new way of analysing the soul; for Winn it was the path to scientifically diagnosing 'abnormalities'; Piddington enlisted Freud's recognition of sexuality in children for her own campaign for sex education.

The second aim of this chapter is to consider one important aspect of psychoanalysis that straddled the philosophical, the therapeutic and the sexual: that of interpreting dreams as a path to the unconscious. These questions have been further prompted after reading a diary by one analysand, B. S. Jones, who records in great detail what he remembers of his dreams. The diary covers a six-month period between 28 November 1929 and 11 June 1930. If Adam Phillips is right in arguing that the 'dream, and its uses, have a history',[4] then how can a document of this sort illuminate the place of psychoanalysis in Australia, suggest how ideas of the unconscious were regarded, and challenge the view that Australian intellectuals have historically been resistant to ideas about inner life?[5]

Furthermore, this diary illuminates a paradox of modernity—that the irrationality of dreams became central to ordering a rational masculine self. Feminist formulations that the 'private and public evolve together' are pertinent to exploring this dimension of modernity.[6] As efficiency, management and the scientific began to define the sexualised self during the interwar years, 'irrational' dream analysis, paradoxically, helped to articulate a rational, sexual identity beyond the private and into the public arena.

Australian 'types'

The Australian national icon of the late nineteenth and early twentieth centuries that had been promoted in literature and popular ballads can be characterised by two distinctive stereotypes: the male pioneer and the bushman. These Australian men embodied the qualities of stoicism, independence, honesty and wholesomeness. In such stereotypes, intimacy was presented as a strain. With the onset of World War I, these qualities were translated into the heroic, mythologised image of the Australian 'digger'.[7] Later the Anzac gave way to the male surfer as the national icon, which became synonymous with unreflective hedonism.[8] While historians have done much to illuminate the class, gender and race assumptions which inform these images,[9] they have often presented Australian culture as lived on the surface with little reflection on inner life.[10] But this did not mean, of course, that there were no efforts at the time to explore interiority.

It was not surprising that in the late 1930s Burgmann would be asked for the name of a good therapist. Known in intellectual circles as the 'Red Bishop' because of his outspoken support of the Soviet Union, Burgmann was a prominent radical thinker and activist. Ordained as an Anglican priest in 1912, he directed his Christian teachings during and after World War I to issues of social justice.[11]

One dimension of his progressive thought was an enthusiasm for Freudian ideas. 'Psychoanalysis', he wrote in 1921, is

> no enemy to religion and philosophy but a distinct gain like all new revelations and facts it tended to broaden and deepen philosophy and religion also . . . the gain to the individual Christian psychologists is very great. An instrument for self-examination is placed in his power such as he [*sic*] never before possessed.[12]

It was through Freud's 'technique . . . which has made the exploration of the human soul possible', that in 'self-analysis for moral and religious purposes and in the light of the Christian ideas we win our way to freedom'. Self-analysis, he claimed, 'should be of untold use to the Christian pastor. When once we have drilled ourselves in self-analysis and better still have been analysed by an expert as well, if such is possible, we find the analysis of other people easier than the analysis of one's self.'[13] Burgmann developed this focus on self-revelation out of a need to connect Christianity to his social concerns.

Ecclesiastical intellectuals were not alone in perceiving the value of ideas relating to the unconscious. Roy Winn was probably the name Burgmann gave to those seeking an analyst whom they could consult. He was the first psychoanalyst to practise in Australia, and a major force behind establishing psychoanalysis in Sydney. Winn enlisted in the Australian Army Medical Corps and served in World War I at Gallipoli, in Egypt and on the Somme. While in London he underwent psychoanalytical training and became a member of the British Psychoanalytical Society. After he returned to Australia, he became Honorary Assistant Physician at Sydney Hospital, but relinquished this post to go into full-time psychoanalytic practice, the first to do so in Australia.[14] His interest in shell-shock victims and the effects of war on the psychology of soldiers endured. In wartime, he asserted, 'the trained psychoanalyst should produce more complete and lasting results, because, in addition to reviving the more superficial causes of inferiority feelings, he [*sic*] aims at relieving deeply buried emotions, such as guilt concerning the impulse to kill'.[15]

During the 1930s Winn published several papers in the *Medical Journal of Australia* advocating the use of psychoanalysis, despite overt antagonism from the medical fraternity. At a meeting of the Medical Science Club in September 1930, he observed that the 'word psychology possesses a constant place in newspaper columns . . . but is seldom found in text books of medicine'. In a discussion which canvassed a number of concepts of Freudian analysis—such as free association, the inferiority complex, and hysteria— Winn argued that medical practitioners could no longer afford to ignore the insights offered by psychology or psychoanalysis.[16] In the future it 'will be considered just as essential', he confidently asserted, 'for medical practitioners to possess a sound knowledge of psychology as of physiology'.[17] For him psychoanalysis was first and foremost a 'method of treatment that can be carried out only by a trained analyst'.[18] In practice, however, the overcrowded and under-resourced asylum system could not easily integrate psychotherapy. With hundreds of patients to attend to, it was impossible for doctors to apply a method that demanded one-to-one treatment.[19]

Feminists joined these debates through considerations of motherhood, sex education, eugenics and birth control. Despite the longstanding antagonism between Freudian ideas and feminism, psychoanalysis has attracted large numbers of female practitioners.[20] The ways in which feminists reconciled the phallocentrism and misogyny with many Freudian ideas is now well documented. In her study of early female psychoanalysts, Nellie Thompson notes that most female psychoanalysts who practised during the interwar years specialised in child analysis or female sexuality.[21] She speculates that there might be 'something in the nature of psychoanalysis itself which women found particularly congenial and attractive'.[22] This trend was also apparent in Australia where women analysts such as Clara Lazar-Geroe and Janet Neild specialised in child psychology.[23]

Marion Piddington, the feminist and eugenicist, supported Freud's views that children were sexual beings.[24] Piddington became an active advocate of eugenic principles towards the end of World War I. As a crusader for sex education, she was well known for her outspoken views on eugenics and promoted sex education as a means to combat venereal disease. In her popular treatise, *Tell Them! The Second Stage of Mothercraft*, published in 1926, Piddington showed how sex education should be made explicit for children. 'Sex-education is now a world-wide movement', she proclaimed, and appealed to parents 'not to blindfold the questioning eyes of growing intelligence, but to set truths before them'.[25] As a eugenicist, her primary concern was the preservation of the race and the need to ensure that women's 'maternal instinct' found full expression. It was the repression of this instinct that Freud had ignored, an omission she identified as a flaw in his analysis. 'The new Psychology', she claimed, 'pays no attention to the subject of maternal repression, the tragedy of which eclipses in its poignant suffering every torment of frustrated human desire.'[26] Piddington connected these arguments to her eugenicist stance, asserting that when women cannot have children they become 'unhinged' and this has severe consequences for 'the certainty of the preservation of the race'.[27]

Middle-class women's magazines reflected this intersection between race and motherhood. While emerging Freudian notions of the self and the emphasis on the emotions were documented, they offered non-psychoanalytic solutions. This reflects the looseness with which psychoanalytic concepts were often used. Until the 1920s the 'unconscious' described 'everything which is not present to consciousness'.[28] These ideas also reflected the Western philosophical tradition which associated the feminine with emotion and the masculine with reason. In the translation to popular usage the analytical, scientific interpretation of the self was lost.

'Nervousness' and 'worry', for instance, figured prominently in the advertisements in the *Everylady's Journal* as mental conditions to be resisted. These were international products translated for a local audience. It was disconcerting the

> worry and fuss we make our imaginary or anticipated ills, which nine times out of ten never happened . . . no one can actually cure us of this habit but ourselves. And if we cannot manage the cure, then strength of mind is sadly lacking. Worrying is due to a mental lack of proportion . . .[29]

Advertisements for Wrigley's chewing gum promised readers that 'the very act of chewing calms the nerves . . . When nerves are calmed, tension is relaxed. The mind is freshened. Concentration is easier.'[30] Advice to mothers was the most striking way in which issues of the emotions were discussed. 'Over anxiety' on the part of the mother 'fosters fear in the child', readers of the *Women's World* were told.[31] 'To deliberately awaken fear in a child', announced *Everylady's Journal*, 'should be treated as a criminal offence. Once aroused, fear is so difficult to quell'.[32] Advice about children was also framed in terms of the unconscious as well as conscious behaviour: 'Be careful to speak correctly', mothers were warned, 'Children copy unconsciously'.[33]

Before psychoanalysis developed as a widespread professional practice in the 1940s, tenets of Freudian ideas were in usage in and outside of the medical arena. Their adoption in Australia at this time was eclectic, and these exchanges offer an alternative to representation of Australian intellectuals as being interested in nationalism and materialism, rather than in questions of inner life. Others sought to apply Freudian concepts more directly to analysing the meaning of the unconscious, and this was especially the case in dream analysis. An understanding of masculine subjectivity through psychoanalytic approaches such as dream interpretation adds another layer to our understanding of masculinity at a time when discourses of scientific management were drawing the expression of sexuality and the self beyond the private and into the public arena.

Dreams

Written in 1900, available in English in 1913, and widely popularised after the war, *The Interpretation of Dreams* sought to explore how meaning could be made from dreams. For Freud, dreams represented the language of the unconscious through condensation and displacement. Condensation refers to the crystallisation of an idea in a single symbol or metaphor. Displacement is when an idea is displaced onto other ideas.[34] There was considerable discussion on these questions by intellectuals in Australia. Burgmann's fascination with psychoanalysis included an abiding interest in Freud's text. He took copious notes from the work, and lectured on it to the working-class men and women who attended his Workers Educational Association classes. In March 1922 he recorded that a 'very good class' of fifty had attended his lecture on dreams.[35]

Another such discussion took place on Aboriginal dreaming. This type of 'dreaming'—where the land is 'seen to embody profound religious and philosophical knowledge' and where memories are conveyed orally through song, art and dance—is a complex and sophisticated method of transmitting cultural knowledge across the generations.[36] In the late nineteenth and early twentieth centuries the dreaming had—as Patrick Wolfe argues— come to be appropriated by anthropologists as a state of stupor experienced by Aboriginal Australians from which they simply needed awakening by white colonials.[37] By the 1930s anthropologists used notions of the psyche to explore the so-called dream-life of Aboriginal people. According to A. P. Elkin, an Anglican priest and anthropologist with close connections to Burgmann, a dream 'to the Aborigines is not a passing fantasy, but a real objective experience in which time and space are no longer obstacles, and in which valuable information and help is gained by the dreamer'.[38] This highlights cultural differences in relation to self-scrutiny, as the confessional mode is noticeably absent from indigenous and non-Western cultures. For instance, as Dipesh Chakrabarty reminds us, since the middle of the nineteenth century Indian novels, letters, diaries and autobiographies 'seldom yield pictures of an endlessly interiorized subject'.[39]

But among white Westerners, writing about dreams is perceived to reveal the self: dreaming, writes Phillips, can be a 'truly solitary form of autobiography'.[40] The diary written by B. S. Jones points to a construction of the modern male self through sexuality and sexual fantasy. Jones was certainly unusual in keeping such a diary, because so few were in therapy at this time. His diary represents an identity in process as fragments of the self are selected, ordered and controlled.[41] While historians have considered the ways in which male subjectivity has been shaped through public discourses, this diary points to a modern male self shaped by taboo and sexual anxiety.

In order to examine this process of the unconscious construction of the male self, I have concentrated on three themes that identify this diary as a modernist text. First, I look at the ordering and recording strategies adopted in this diary; second, I consider what aspects of his life occupied Jones's mental and emotional self; and finally, I look at the role the analyst was to have played in the process of defining and 'curing' the self.

Ordering and recording: emotional management

During the 1920s and 1930s the very act of writing and documenting one's dreams revealed a desire to contain an irrational and illusory world. This is not to say that people did not have dreams before they had the mechanisms through which to analyse them, but that there was a discernible shift to making the self understood through adopting the scientific approach of dream analysis. As Zygmut Baumann has noted, this desire to order is a 'modern' inclination. 'Among the multitude of impossible tasks that modernity set itself', he argues, 'the task of order . . . stands out'.[42] Dreams become ordered according to linear time, not ill defined through fragmentary time. Thus the management of emotions became an important part of the need to ensure order in society. In an article in the *Sydney Morning Herald* in July 1935, Kenneth Henderson encapsulated the need to discipline the emotions. The management of emotions, he argued, would 'add to the value, the efficiency, the harmony, and the health of our living'. Furthermore, it was important to 'discipline emotion to the service of judgement' by avoiding 'orgies of emotion. Do not wallow in grief, disappointment, sensuality, anger or what not'.[43]

Jones's diary was written at a time when dreaming was perceived to be an important aspect of understanding the self, managing it and defining it. Memory is part of dream life, but can it be willed? 'Some little dream activity', records Jones one December night: 'woke up and determined to remember details; on getting up find cannot remember a single detail'.[44] For his entry on 30 November the diarist notes that he is 'dimly aware of having had several dreams but details too vague to permit recall. After dreaming—whilst still asleep—I am semi-consciously aware of [the] necessity of re-membering all dreams with as [much] detail as possible.'[45] Throughout the diary he is determined to remember his dreams. 'Woke up and determined to remember details', he writes with some frustration in December 1929, but 'on getting-up find cannot remember a single detail'.[46] In the history of dream analysis, the ordering of dreams for meanings of the self reflects the modernist, scientific project of management and order.

Emotional life

What preoccupies Jones's mental and emotional world? Sexuality figures significantly in his inner life. His virility is part of his masculine identity, and his documentation of details of dreaming of particular sexual encounters suggest an acquaintance with Freud's writings:

> I find myself in a room with a young woman; she is a sensible and reasonable girl . . . She readily agrees to sexual intercourse & this we proceed to carry out. I question her if she desires me to deploy a contraceptive device which I have in my possession . . . She replied in the negative whereupon I gladly cast the device to one side. I was tempted to have connection with her right away, but on second thoughts decided to postpone actual intercourse until after some preliminary 'wooing'. Waking up at this point, I realised that (although I did not recognised her as such in my dream) the girl was my own sister.[47]

Sexuality was central to Freudian understandings of the self. Angus McLaren argues that by explaining that all neuroses had a 'sexual origin', Freud appeared 'to give order to a disorderly world'.[48] For Freud, 'un-conscious sexual wishes provided the motivating force for dreams'.[49] In the diary there are descriptions of taboo activities—such as incest, homosexual-ity, bigamy, adultery, sex with an older woman—and of betrayal and deceit. If dreams are about what is unacceptable, disagreeable, or shameful, then Jones's dreams are revelations of the taboo sexual topics of the day.[50] Anxiety plays a crucial role in dreaming for, as Ruth Bers Shapiro writes, it is both 'a response to unacceptable wishes *and* serves to disguise them'.[51] Hence Jones writes of how he dreamt of a 'number of boys, including myself each occupying a separate bed, in a long dormitory. Each boy engaged in experimenting with a clip device attached to his penis'.[52] Of sexual deceit, he notes: 'Am sitting with Miss J . . . I put my arm around her waist; she rather resents this at first. Later however she seems to quite enjoy our "kissing and cuddling". At the time I am somewhat afraid that E will enter and discover us'.[53] The taboo is stressed in his accounts as he dreams of having an 'improvised affair—rough and ready'.[54]

During the 1920s and 1930s open debate about sex management and sex education created an opportunity for much discussion.[55] The approach towards understanding sex became more scientific and rational, with an emphasis on psychology, although sex was still considered primarily for procreation.[56] The diary entries carry the hallmark of this sexual openness and signal a shift towards discussion of the private in public, a cultural and social change encouraged by discussions of Freud's theories on sexuality.

The role of the analyst

The paradox of this diary is that while it is a record of one person's inner-most thoughts and feelings, usually kept private, it is meant to be read by an expert. Writing for analysis by such an expert shapes the narrative in the diary. Jones's therapist figures in his dreams and he provides details of his encounters with him. In this document it is the analyst, not the dream itself, which holds the key to understanding the unconscious. At this time there was a reliance on the expert to help in understanding the mysteries of dreams. Jones reveals a belief in the interpretative powers of the expert in documenting these dreams. In his dreams the analyst is shown to cure him of his ills. Mr X:

> is seeking to find the cause of my trouble in twisting and turning my body about in all sorts of ways ... Mr. X is working very energetically & despite several failures, seems determined to discover the cause of the trouble. After a brief while, he places my body in such a position that my back is bent and my hands somehow get entangled in a knot ... I am now cured.[57]

On another occasion he wishes to please his therapist and tells him what he wishes to hear:

> Next I find myself talking to Mr X, inform him that despite the fact that I am still much of a sinner, am desirous of entering the Christian ministry (this statement was not altogether sincere as it was made mainly for the purpose of pleasing X). He replies that it is doubtful if I will be able to study under him as he is about to be transferred somewhere else.[58]

In this diary there is a self-conscious effort to order the workings of the unconscious. It is meant for an audience—his analyst—and the diarist's sense of self is shaped in an interactive way with the analyst, especially when the information that emerges through an analysis of a dream is often integrated into subsequent dreams.[59] Despite any doubts Jones may express consciously or unconsciously about his role, his diary reflects the key place the analyst was thought to have had in the 'curing' process.

Nancy Schnog argues that in a 'cultural history of emotional life', the emotions are 'historically contingent, socially specific and politically situated'.[60] Such a history looks at 'the reasons why . . . psychological concepts . . . gain cultural authority and lose explanatory power at particular historical moments'.[61] The analysis of dreams preoccupied intellectuals during the interwar period, and prior to the professionalisation of psychoanalysis in Australia, such ideas were discussed and contested in various quarters. It is paradoxical that at a time when the rational was prioritised, it was the irrational that was seen as holding the key to understanding the rational mind. The urge to document one's dreams in a systematic fashion reflected the modern Western desire to manage, control and scientifically order society.

By drawing on a diary of dreams, we can discern the influence of Freudian analysis in the understandings of the self amongst some Australian intellectuals. During the interwar period, the contemporary public discussion of sexuality in the public arena provided the space within which to articulate these issues. The examination of interior life, as explored both in this diary by B. S. Jones and in discussions by intellectuals, implies a challenge to the familiar representation of Australian masculinity as unconditionally resistant to questions of interiority. While popular magazines could flippantly suggest that 'nervousness' could be cured by non-psychoanalytic techniques like taking a cup of cocoa or chewing gum, for others the chaos and fragmentation of their dreams paradoxically offered them the key to ordering their neuroses.

3

History, psychoanalysis, modernism

kylie valentine

THERE ARE A number of possibilities when it comes to considering the terms 'psychoanalysis' and 'history'. Psychoanalysis tells individual and cultural histories. It emerged at a particular historical moment, and its doctrines have particular things to say about the forces and importance of history. Equally, there are a number of ways to historicise psychoanalysis. Psychoanalysis emerged from such things as *fin de siècle* Vienna, the crisis of religion, the ascendancy of science, the prospect of revolution, and other concepts of similar size and manageability. From the perspective of a certain kind of intellectual history, or a certain awareness of current intellectual concerns, the real or imagined decline of psychoanalysis suggests another way of historicising it. Increasingly marginal to psychiatry, psychoanalysis has also been targeted as outmoded in critical theory. If it emerged as both a therapeutic technique and a cultural narrative, psychoanalysis is perhaps a historical presence in both fields. The best way of understanding psychoanalysis and history, in other words, may be to consider psychoanalysis as part of history.

If so, there is a link between this decline of psychoanalysis and postmodernism. As weighty and complicated a term as psychoanalysis, postmodernism cannot be considered in any detail here. I think it reasonably uncontroversial, though, to nominate Gilles Deleuze and Felix Guattari as important to it, and to connect them to critiques of psychoanalysis. Indebted as they were to psychoanalysis, Deleuze and Guattari nonetheless spent a fair amount of time excoriating it, and post-psychoanalytic theories of subjectivity bear the mark of their influence. Deleuze especially is also associated with another postmodern preoccupation, that of interdisciplinarity. Postmodernism has brought about the recognition that new types of knowledge and new ways of organising them are necessary. In universities today interdisciplinarity is often promoted as a novel set of epistemological foundations and objects of knowledge. Paul Bové is among those who identify Deleuze with these new exigencies and knowledges, seeing Deleuze as occupying an 'ironically and historically critical position on his own disciplinary formation so that he might then confidently cut across it all'.[1]

There is nothing particularly rash about discussing the decline of psychoanlaysis as coeval with modernism's successor. Neither is it especially original to connect psychoanalysis with modernism. Modernism and psychoanalysis are regarded as products of the same processes, arising from the same cultural quakes. Sometimes modernism is understood as emerging from new narratives of a new world, of which psychoanalysis is one. From this perspective, modernism is responsive to 'the scenario of our chaos', consequent to 'Heisenberg's "Uncertainty principle", of the destruction of civilisation and reason in the First World War, of the world changed and reinterpreted by Marx, Freud, and Darwin'.[2] Sometimes cause and effect are seen as the reverse of this, such that the conjunction of early twentieth-century art and science produced psychoanalysis, which becomes 'the point where the biological metaphors of late nineteenth-century thought met the genuinely modern demand for a science of man'.[3]

Either way the aesthetic practices and thematic concerns critically important to modernism—decentring of the subject, crises in narratives of the self, biological and scientific knowledges, classicism, sexuality, embodiment—are also those of psychoanalysis. Auden's 'we are all Freudians now' recalls the importance of psychoanalysis to interwar culture as well as to the personal networks of some English moderns. Virginia Woolf's brother Adrian was a psychoanalyst; her friends James and Alix Strachey were Freud's translators; the Woolfs' Hogarth Press published those translations. Psychoanalysis presented a program for radical cultural upheaval and a nexus of modern scientific discourses: think of Emma Goldman at Freud's lectures, or the anthropologist Bronislaw Malinowski at a meeting of the British Psycho-Analytic Society.

Psychoanalysis also emerged, with modernism, from the conditions of imperialism and is, with modernism, a utopian, universalising project. The revolutionary energies of both are inseparable from their limitations. Loss of these energies, and of master narratives like modernism and psycho-analysis, are central to postmodern thought. What I want to suggest here is that another concept central to postmodernism, interdisciplinarity, is present at the making of psychoanalysis and modernism. The history of psycho-analysis is only rarely considered in postmodern critiques of it, and the history of interdisciplinarity only rarely acknowledged. Psychoanalysis and modernist literature were necessarily involved with several disciplines, and all make for discouraging reading. Democratic protestations disguise, often poorly, radically anti-democratic impulses. Breathtaking misogyny and racism appear frequently in unexpected as well as obvious places. The capacity for knowledge and understanding is denied to all but a select few. Optimistic and confident theories about the sources and treatments of mental distress juxtapose with consistent failure to relieve that distress.

Perhaps not only the pessimistic occasionally notice these elements recurring in contemporary literature, science and commentary. Beyond noting the problems of the modernist era, and noting that these problems remain unsolved, it may be worthwhile acknowledging the antecedents of contemporary interdisciplinarity. Analysis of the particular locations of psychoanalysis, the impact of psychoanalysis on other kinds of knowledge and representation, and the ways in which discourses of the self intersect across modernist science and art do not reveal any compelling reasons to defend it from criticism. What this analysis does reveal is that much of the imperialist reach of psychoanalysis so distasteful to contemporary readers—refusal of situated knowledges and contingency, claims to universalism—is the *product* of interdisciplinary formation. Neglect of this interdisciplinarity in contemporary interdisciplinary criticism is ironic, and perhaps nothing more than ironic. But if psychoanalysis is nearing the limits of its use to critical theory, then its history should be acknowledged, and the meanings of its interdisciplinarity should, perhaps, serve as a caution.

Interdisicplinary histories

Both psychoanalysis and modernism are sometimes viewed in terms of ahistorical wilfulness and hubris, as self-constructed as outside of history. Freud, famously, anointed himself heir to Copernicus and Darwin, naming the emergence of psychoanalysis as the third 'injury suffered by mankind's self-love' after the two scientific revolutions bearing their names.[4] The utopian tendencies in both psychoanalysis and modernism can be under-stood with varying degrees of forgiveness, and the prominence given to the 'universal' and the 'timeless' in modernist and psychoanalytic texts has been the subject of feminist and other criticism. The preoccupations of modernist and psychoanalytic practitioners with the importance of the individual genius and with the novelty and transformative potential of their own work must appear to most contemporary eyes as anachronistic and deluded. To most contemporary eyes also, the emergence of psychoanalysis and modernism has much less to do with individual geniuses and novelty than with specific institutional and historical processes. A number of critics have in fact argued that modernism especially could only have emerged the way it did because of these processes. Psychoanalysis, especially Anglophone psychoanalysis, has not been subject to the same degree of study. Yet if the arguments made about modernism's history are applied to psychoanalysis, the relationship between them is illuminated in new ways.

One of the best known of such historical accounts of literary modernism is Perry Anderson's conceptualisation of a field of force triangulated by three coordinates.[5] If Anderson's model is applied to psychoanalysis, a similar field can be mapped. The first of these is the 'imaginative proximity of social revolution', brought about by feminist and working-class mobilisation and transformations in class relations. Texts such as Freud's *The Future of an Illusion* and *Civilisation and its Discontents* have long been recognised as psychoanalytic responses to social turmoil, and Freud's responses to feminism and attitudes to women are foundationally important to the practical and theoretical bases of classical psychoanalysis.

Anderson's second coordinate of modernism is 'the still incipient, hence essentially *novel*, emergence of the key technologies or inventions of the second industrial revolution: telephone, radio, automobile, aircraft and so on'. Technologies of communication were influential in the formation of psychoanalytic theory and practice—it is not for nothing that psychoanalysis is known as the talking cure. Interest in the mechanical and new technologies is much more visible in art and literature than in psychoanalysis; nevertheless, the impact of modernisation and technology on the individual consciousness and on the organisation of culture was important to psychoanalytic doctrine. More broadly, psychoanalysis emerged from, and contributed to, cultural imaginings of an era of scientific advance and social transformation.

Anderson's third coordinate, the most interesting for our purposes, is the 'codification of a highly formalised *academicism* in the visual and other arts', foregrounding the emergence of literature as a discipline as important to modernist production. Psychoanalysis is not an academic discipline, but disciplinarity was an important force in its emergence and development. More particularly, interdisciplinarity was an important force, although it had an impact at odds with the claims made for interdisciplinarity today. Through the 1920s and 1930s writers and reviewers in the *International Journal of Psycho-analysis* found nothing that could not be explained by the proper application of psychoanalytic principles: the development of neurotic symptoms, the symbolism of clothes, the writings of Plato, the kinship behaviour of 'primitives'. This kind of epistemological sweep seems to be at odds with particular, located knowledge, and the journal itself proclaims the need for psychoanalysis to be adopted as a master narrative at every turn. Yet, as Judith Ryan points out, this global project of emergent psycho-analysis is neither isolated nor inexplicable. What appears to us now to be psychoanalysts overstepping their disciplinary bounds of psychology or psychiatry can be comprehended in terms of the interconnectedness of psychology and philosophy in the eighteenth and nineteenth centuries. Early psychologists' concerns would be understood today as philosophical and their thinking was indebted to philosophical traditions: 'arguing against nineteenth-century positivism they attempted to revive in newly modified form ideas that had been espoused in the eighteenth century by Berkeley, Hume, and Locke'.[6]

Early psychology looked a lot like philosophy, which goes some way to explaining why early psychologists argued about things that would not now be understood as psychology's business. Psychoanalysis was interpreted in some quarters as one of many new psychologies, an interpretation that provided an additional challenge to psychoanalysts. The British Psycho-Analytic Association was formed in 1913. The London-based *International Journal of Psycho-analysis* was the official organ of the association from 1920. Both association and journal were from the outset concerned explicitly with several tasks: the dissemination of Freud's work in English; the struggle for leadership over the New York association in introducing psychoanalysis to the Anglophone world; and the successful promotion of psychoanalysis as a medical science to the medical scientific community. However, the biggest perceived challenge to the British association was the emergence of other new psychologies, especially the work of the eclectics at places like the Tavistock Institute and Craiglockhart Military Hospital. The first issue of the *Journal* featured an editorial by Ernest Jones arguing that opposition to psychoanalysis, especially in the United States, had taken an insidious turn in the form of

> acquiescence in the new ideas on the condition that their value is discounted, the logical consequences not drawn from them, and their meaning diluted until it may be regarded as 'harmless' . . . under all sorts of specious guises and by the aid of various seductive catchwords or principles entirely legitimate in themselves, such as 'resistance to dogma', 'freedom of thought', 'widening of vision' and so on.[7]

English reticence to discuss sex, English anti-Semitism and English anti-Teutonic feeling were all recognised as obstacles. But the greatest threat to psychoanalysis in England was, at least as far as leading practitioners and acolytes were concerned, the dilution of psychoanalytic ideas and the selective taking up of psychoanalytic practices. Psychoanalysis needed to be accepted in its entirety, or the strength of its ideas would be lost. Freud's insights would not survive if they were absorbed into the broad discipline of psychology.

Interdisciplinarity was important to the formation of psychology, and to the struggles of psychoanalysts to maintain the autonomy of their practice. The interdisciplinary formation of these fields provides a partial explanation for the claims made on behalf of psychoanalysis, and other cultural and scientific interwar discourses. Psychoanalysis emerged from struggles over the right to explain the self, and at a moment when transformation of both self and society seemed imminent. A medical, psychological self emerged from nineteenth-century literature and philosophy, and became the particular province of the new scientific discipline of psychology. Protestations made by psychoanalysts that psychoanalysis was certainly not one among many new psychologies can be comprehended in terms of this development. It was seen as necessary to stake out territory, to make efforts so that psychoanalysis was not weakened.

Perry Anderson's model of literary modernism is helpful to understanding psychoanalysis. On face value it suggests only that the same forces produced them both. Yet the connections between them are clearly more developed than those of context. It is possible to extend the question of disciplinarity to include literature. Michael Levenson's genealogy of modernism, for example, argues that the secularising of society in the nineteenth century is reflected in the importance of the individual consciousness to modernist literature. He argues that religion is not replaced with morality or aesthetics; instead 'they came to be translated into psychological terms without losing their force'.[8] Literature too, then, was concerned with the new discipline of psychology, and itself became a discipline at around the same time. The historical formation of psychoanalysis and modernist literature reveals shared concerns, and shared demands. More than this, as the next section will show, history was an important, shared element of the way both were written.

Histories of the self

Arguments with modernism and psychoanalysis about the lack of historical perspective in both make most sense in the context of discussions of institutions or movements. While accepting that preoccupations with the timeless and universal do represent an ahistorical streak in both fields, I have tried to suggest that the ahistoricism of both can be understood in terms other than that of individuals' arrogance. However, even a cursory examination of some of the most well-known modernist and psychoanalytic texts reveals that the question of history is a shared formal concern of both. In other words, even if both the modernist and psychoanalytic *fields* share assumptions or claims about being outside or beyond the forces of history, these forces nonetheless remain a shared concern of their *texts*.

History for Freud and modernist writers is, unsurprisingly, discussed with reference to the individual and often addressed through an examination of memory, generation, or lived time. Many of Freud's best-known texts, in fact, are concerned with the history of individuals and the history of social organisation more than anything else: *Totem and Taboo*; *Moses and Monotheism*; the case histories; the essays on sexuality. In some ways there could be no more obvious argument than that psychoanalysis is concerned with history, but in other ways this argument is too simplistic to be of much use. For history in the psychoanalytic economy is a fraught and complex force, and both of these attributes were illuminated during the 1980s and 1990s by the controversies generated by the work of Jeffrey Masson. His *The Assault on Truth* argues that Freud's work with hypnosis in the late years of the nineteenth century made him aware of the widespread extent of child sexual abuse. Unable to countenance this, and through a failure of personal and professional courage, Freud changed his story. Modifying his 'seduction' theory to the subsequently vital model of fantasy, Freud unceremoniously dropped the political hot potato of child assault. Rather than childhood abuse being a traumatic *reality* for his patients, those patients were instead describing their childhood *fantasies* of sexual encounters with their parents.[9] The impact of the text was spectacular. Masson was sacked as curator of the Freud Archives and more than one reviewer suggested that book and author should be consigned to oblivion.

John Forrester, however, in one of the more nuanced responses to Masson's work, argues that Freud did not necessarily decide that he was wrong when he hypothesised sexual assault as the cause of adult trauma. Rather, what 'he focused on was the fact that it was *memories* of these events that were of significance to him as a neurologist-psychotherapist'.[10] The reality of the event was less important to Freud than the memory of it, argues Forrester, because it is the memory of trauma that causes conflict within an individual, and this conflict is the target of psychoanalytic therapy. The novelty of Freud's theorising comes through the argument that the process of remembering is an essential mediation between trauma and neurosis; without this process, the empirically verifiable evidence of the trauma is not sufficient to effect neurosis. On the other hand, the memory of trauma will be sufficient to effect a neurosis regardless of the empirical evidence of the trauma remembered. After his decision that traumatic memories of early childhood did not lend themselves to a retrospective splitting of reality from fantasy, Freud established a therapeutic contract where his patients' testimonies were trusted as genuine, but the reality of the events they described was not regarded as relevant. Forrester argues that Freud disregarded the distinction between fantasy and reality, trusting what his patients said without deciding whether the events were real or not: 'The event was now bracketed off, with its reality-sign ... regarded as an added feature, rather like quotation marks in the written reporting of speech'.[11]

There are clearly problems with this, most obviously those raised by the decision to treat someone as an unreliable witness to the reality of their own life. Nevertheless, the argument that psychoanalysis is concerned with the lived history of an event rather than the empirical evidence of it, with its psychic impact rather than objectively assessed effects, suggests that complex processes of history are important not only to psychoanalytic therapeutic practice, but to the formation of the psychoanalytic self. Freud's 'bracketing' of the actual event also reveals that classical psychoanalysis is concerned with the nature of experience and its 'reality' and the importance of narrative to self-construction, concerns often associated with more contemporary critical theory.

History and the lived experience of history are also crucial to modernist texts and doctrine. Again the importance of history is in many ways easy to detect and obvious to argue. T. S. Eliot's emphasis on tradition and Ezra Pound's interest in classicism are well known, and point to a certain understanding of history within important strands of modernist doctrine.[12] The argument that some modernists thought that they could escape history through force of will has some merit, but it should be recalled also that access to knowledge of history was for these modernists an essential precondition for the production of literature. Like Freud, modernists such as Pound, Eliot and H. D. were concerned with the historical links between interwar European society and the ancient civilisations of Greece and Rome that were then, as now, understood as its heritage. Other modernists like Conrad and Eliot (again) shared Freud's interest in the historical ruptures and discontinuities between interwar European society and the 'primitive' societies of Africa and the Pacific that were then, as now, understood as being connected to the former only in evolutionary terms.[13]

However, we can also see important links between psychoanalytic and modernist representations of history in the attention both paid to the experience of history, to lived time. Virginia Woolf's published works reveal a consistent concern with temporality, and her 1925 novel *Mrs Dalloway* is critically regarded as the novel in which the lived time of consciousness is most successfully conveyed. The novel is told over the course of a single day, recounting the childhood and more immediate histories of its two protagonists: the eponymous Clarissa Dalloway, and a former soldier, Septimus Smith, who is psychically distressed by the effects of war, and suicides towards the novel's close. Several different time frames are represented; the importance of memory and history to the present of each character is constantly evoked. It is, among other things, the traumatic memory of war and the intrusion of the past into the present that clearly disturbs Smith. For Smith, Dalloway and the novel's other characters, present identities are more than simply the product of their histories; their histories are an episodic, significant presence. *Mrs Dalloway* shares with Woolf's other novels a challenge to linear temporality and the narratives of patrilineal genealogy. Her writing, like Freud's, reveals a concern with the importance of memory in the making of the self, as well as underlining the traumatic potential of memory.

Woolf's work and life have been the subjects of a great deal of contemporary feminist criticism, and this criticism reveals a further complication to the relationships between modernism, postmodernism and psychoanalysis. She suffered mental distress throughout her life, and this distress has been linked to her experience of sexual assault perpetrated by her two stepbrothers. Biographies of Woolf have been constructed around different interpretations of what that assault was, and what it meant to her. The presence of psychoanalysis in contemporary critical and literary theory should be acknowledged here, for Freud's bracketing of empirical evidence in the search for an experiential truth is certainly a point of origin for current thinking on situated knowledge and contested realities. Classical psychoanalysis would have been no help to Woolf, and she was rightly critical of some of its mechanisms and assumptions. Yet powerful feminist readings of Woolf's sexual trauma argue that the empirical evidence presented by defenders of her stepbrothers—of minimal bodily damage, of the brevity or small number of assaults—is beside the point. It does not matter who thinks the assaults on her were trivial: she did not.[14] The memory of that assault caused her distress and informed her narratives of self all her life. These readings then resemble Freud's revised theory in significant ways. Jeffrey Masson has been an influential critic of psychoanalysis, and the violence done by psychoanalysts to patients' histories have been important to feminist critiques. Here and elsewhere, the ambivalent functions of psychoanalysis are not easily resolved.

More generally, it can be seen that some of the most important and obvious concerns of modernism and psychoanalysis were shared by them. The impact of history, of the remote and exotic, can be detected in the consciousness of a single individual, and an individual consciousness is the most productive site for any analysis of history. Language is crucial to the formation of the self, and new narratives are needed to capture the reality of experience. Freud famously argued that hysterics can make no 'smooth' histories of themselves; Virginia Woolf used the same word in rejecting the existing conventions of literary narrative. Unacknowledged and hidden psychic forces were treated as more interesting than visible actions, and conflict between individuals was often explained in terms of conflict within them. Those narratives of history that seemed to fit these projects, especially anthropology, were negotiated and interpreted. Those that didn't, most obviously Marxist and socialist histories, were largely ignored.

Conclusion

At a time when both psychoanalysis and modernism are often described as constituting, yet being superseded by, our own moment, connections between the two movements may seem of historical interest, but little more. Were this the case, then these connections would still, I hope, be worth elaborating. They reveal the traffic across distinct terrains of formative concepts, ideas, and ideologies; they make visible the impact of science on literature, and of literature on science. It is not always possible to see the mutual influences and interdependencies of contemporary cultural and scientific discourses, and the extent of mutual influence on two of the most important discourses of the twentieth century is striking.

Beyond this, however, I want to suggest that the historical connections between modernism and psychoanalysis, and their shared concerns with particular forces of history reveal broader questions. I will mention only two. First, the impact of discipline formation and interdisciplinarity on psychoanalysis and modernism—neither of which are disciplines themselves—suggests that the contemporary place of interdisciplinary and cross-disciplinary study within universities has unacknowledged antecedents. It suggests also that those characteristics of classical psychoanalysis and modernism most distasteful to contemporary discourses of interdisciplinarity may be a function of the interdisciplinarity of both. For it can be seen that much of the rhetoric of the timeless and universal, much of the imperialist reach of modernism and psychoanalysis, was produced in part by the exigencies of discipline formation. Analogously, much of the postmodern concern with the interdisciplinary and institutional nomadism refers to the importance of acknowledging the contingent and situated—the particularity of knowledge. Contemporary preoccupations with the interdisciplinary repudiate the consequences of a historical instance of interdisciplinarity. This suggests a neglect of the history of discourses of the self.

Second, the shared, complex narratives of history in psychoanalysis and modernism suggest that the novelties of post-psychoanalytic theories of subjectivity and postmodern literature may also be overstated. Both psycho-analysis and Anglophone modernism have been categorised as master nar-ratives in some discussions of postmodernism; the impact of Deleuze on most theories of subjectivity and the emergence of postcolonial literature have been distinct but complementary forces in the problematising of both. Again, those currents within both movements that lend themselves most to such designations are illuminated by historical analysis. However, analysis of modernism and psychoanalysis by postmodern scholars also reveals emphases on memory and history, and emphases on those aspects most often associated with postmodernism: unreliability and fragmentation; ex-perience and its availability to language; trauma; the embodied self. While other chapters in this book defend ably by exemplification the uses of psychoanalysis to contemporary writing, it is occasionally worth offering a more concrete, institutional explication of the histories of modernism and psychoanalysis.

4

The inner and outer world of queer life

Robert Reynolds

ESPITE A CENTURY of psychoanalytic research and writing, not to mention
practice, using psychoanalysis in academic work remains a risky proposition. I was reminded of this recently when discussing a grant proposal
with my university's Director of Research Development. A formidable character, with a daunting reputation for grooming successful applicants and
puncturing the egos of longwinded academics, she winced when she came
across the word 'psychoanalysis' in the draft of my grant application. 'Can't
we get rid of this?', she inquired, 'It will win you no friends'.

Psychoanalysis, leaving aside the optimism of some of its tamer North
American variants, was never meant to win friends and influence people,
but it can still come as something of a shock to find how thoroughly unsettling academics find any mention of the psychoanalytic, especially in the
English-speaking world. There are exceptions of course. Universities in
Britain and North America do run well-established courses in psychoanalysis
—its practice, theory and application to social, political and cultural
research. The British, in particular, have developed a reputation for rigorous
psychoanalytic readings of political and cultural formations. Writers like
Janet Sayers, Michael Rustin, Barry Richards, R. D. Hinshelwood, Jacqueline
Rose, Christopher Bollas and the frighteningly prolific Adam Phillips cross
easily from clinical theory into psychoanalytically informed social analysis.
In Australia, however, psychoanalysis as a designated field of academic
study is less common, with once flourishing centres of psycho-social

analysis, like The University of Melbourne's Politics Department, no longer pre-eminent.

It is true that locally psychoanalysis has moved obliquely into English and cultural studies departments. The recent linguistic turn in the humanities has paved the way for psychoanalytic reading of literary texts and popular culture. But even in this growth field, only a particular brand of psychoanalysis seems to hold sway. With its emphasis upon language as the entry into subjectivity, Lacanian theory has proved especially attractive for textual theorists. Jacques Lacan's devotees may well see themselves as the true inheritors of Freud, sometimes shamelessly so, but a healthy self-image and good public relations should not be mistaken for copyright. Psychoanalysis in the twenty-first century is a very broad church. The followers of Freud, Lacan, Melanie Klein, Donald Winnicott and Heinz Kohut, to name the most obvious schools, can all lay claim to the mantle of psychoanalysis. My point is that in the academic world of Australian literary and cultural theory you would hardly know this. Freud and French psychoanalysis reign supreme.

But at least psychoanalysis is seen as a valid tool by literary and cultural theorists. Moving further afield into political science, history and the social sciences, psychoanalytically informed research still struggles for legitimacy. Many political scientists, historians and social scientists—most perhaps—continue to view psychoanalysis with suspicion. The list of common objections to the deployment of psychoanalysis in political biography that Judith Brett outlines in this volume could be extended to the general critique of psychoanalytically informed research. It is claimed that psychoanalysis is ahistorical or too universalistic, both immediate disqualifications in an age of modest research goals. For others, psychoanalysis is too historically specific, an intriguing product of late nineteenth-century bourgeois sexual repression that is of little relevance in today's sexually liberal world. This last objection—that psychoanalysis is all about sex and the repression of drives—is especially galling for those of us who have kept abreast of psychoanalytic theory since Freud's death in 1939. While Lacanians have turned from instincts to language, psychoanalysts in England and America have replaced the primacy of drives with an emphasis upon unconscious fantasy, relationships, attachments and the self. In fact, the shift to object relations, self-objects and intersubjectivity in contemporary English-speaking psychoanalysis has led some commentators to fear that sex is dropping out altogether from the psychoanalytic schema.[1] So much for the dominance of sex-obsessed Freudians!

A more sophisticated set of critics view psychoanalysis as too implicated in a normative discourse of modernity to be of much use for we ironic postmoderns. Such an approach is strongly favoured in my own field, gay/

queer history and sociology. Here the hand of Michel Foucault is felt, perhaps more heavily than he intended. I'll return to Foucault and his followers below. For the moment, suffice to say that it is the brave queer historian or sociologist who ventures into the academic arena with psychoanalysis in his or her tool kit. It is not that all queer theorists are hostile to psychoanalysis. Queer textual theorists are not averse to citing Freud and Lacan as they read the melancholic shadow of homosexuality into the most heterosexual of texts. Social theorist Leo Bersani has drawn brilliantly upon Freud to explain how with AIDS, the normal fear of male homosexuality has been promoted to 'a compelling terror as a secret fantasy becomes a public spectacle: the spectacle of men dying from . . . the suicidal ecstasy of taking their sex like a woman'.[2] Of late, even the work of that most clinical of analysts, Melanie Klein, has begun to attract interest. Philosopher Judith Butler, revered by many queer theorists, has picked up on Klein's account of melancholia to flesh out the psychic paradox of subjection.[3] Butler's previous work on the performance of gender owed something of a debt to Joan Riviere's psychoanalytic writing during the 1920s on the masquerade of gender, notably her 1929 article 'Womanliness as a masquerade'.[4] But for the most part queer historians and sociologists are holding firm against psychoanalytic incursions, past and present.

Giving psychoanalytically informed papers to an audience of historians and sociologists is thus a bracing experience. In America, that bastion of the psychoanalytic establishment, queer historians are particularly dismissive of psychoanalysis. A look of pity crosses their face when you mention Freud; of incomprehension if you cite Klein, Winnicott or Kohut. Question time can be tricky. Women's studies graduates will point out impatiently that Freud was patriarchal, nominating Freud's case study of Dora as conclusive and final evidence. Those who have read Jeffrey Masson or Alice Miller will suggest you are denying the tragedy of child abuse. Poststructuralists will chide you for deploying a normalising discourse. And sometimes, appropriately enough, the mere mention of psychoanalysis flushes out the eccentric. 'What of Prozac?', I was once asked. Did I support the use of antidepressants that were purported to have severe side effects? ('In your case, sir', I was tempted to reply, 'most certainly'.)

Against these claims, I want to stake a place for psychoanalysis in the study of queer life. Psychoanalysis is important, I believe, because it attempts to join, not always successfully, the inner and outer world of individuals and groups. This is not to set up a simple division between inner and outer with psychoanalysis as some sort of exclusive drawbridge. Indeed, an enduring legacy of psychoanalysis is an appreciation of the dynamic relationship between the internal and the external life of individuals, groups, and even nations. It may be the case that the further psychoanalysis moves away from the individual the more speculative its 'findings', but this need not be construed as a failing. Psychoanalytically informed research will always be speculative. How could it be otherwise when psychoanalysis is the art of speculation, despite Freud's ambitions for a psychoanalytic science? In its better moments, psychoanalysis tries to skirt both a psychic determinism (whether drive or fantasy, symbolic or relational) and a reading of history that reduces subjectivity to a simple process of socialisation. It's a precarious and imperfect balancing act, but at least it is an act that psychoanalysis attempts to stage.

This chapter will look specifically at how accounts of psychoanalysis and homosexuality have interacted and clashed. This is a large topic which must be dealt with here briefly and selectively. I'll begin by surveying how psychoanalysis has imagined homosexuality over the last century, and then turn to the more recent deployment and critique of psychoanalysis by post gay liberation theorists of homosexuality. As we shall see, for the most part psychoanalysis and homosexuality have had an unhappy relationship. A closer analysis, however, reveals a relationship of some mutual dependence. In my concluding section, I'll compare a psychoanalytic and a non-psychoanalytic reading of queer sexual practice, and argue for an approach to sexuality that can encompass, but not merge, both.

Homosexuality and the history of psychoanalysis

That psychoanalysis and homosexuality retain an uneasy relationship, despite some recent compromises, was evident at the Fortieth Congress of the International Psychoanalytical Association in 1997. A panel discussion on 'Sexuality in the age of AIDS' quickly collapsed into a heated debate on the perverse tendencies of male homosexuality. Argument flowed between those analysts attempting to 'defuse the block about homosexuality/perversion' and those for whom the link between homosexuality and perversion remained all too evident. Just as one analyst argued that homosexuality was not by definition a perversion, and that the classification of perversion be reserved for 'compulsions marked by a taste for destructive pleasure', another analyst moved to fill the gap.[5] Psychoanalysis had promised that the liberation of sexuality would cultivate more empathic relationships between men and women, lamented a defender of the homosexuality/perversion nexus, but instead 'what we have today after a hundred years of psychoanalysis is an enormous quantity of homosexuals', many of whom were now infected with AIDS.[6] It was a novel twist to the debate—that psychoanalysis was actually encouraging perversion and sickness—but it encapsulated the emotive tenor of the discussion. There was a 'visceral atmosphere throughout the discussion', admitted the panel reporters, 'with much work to be done, not only with regard to the psycho-analytic institution but in each analyst, about his own prejudices and attitudes'.[7]

It should come as no surprise that homosexuality prompts such analytic uneasiness. Since the death of Freud, the history of the relationship between psychoanalysis and homosexuality has been one of mutual distrust, if not loathing. Yet as historian Henry Abelove has demonstrated, Freud took a consistently liberal approach to homosexuality throughout his career. In his much-cited 1935 letter to the American mother of a homosexual, Freud wrote that while homosexuality was no advantage, 'it is nothing to be ashamed of, no vice, no degradation, it cannot be classified as an illness, we consider it to be a variation of the sexual function produced by a certain arrest of sexual development'.[8] As early as 1903 Freud had argued that homosexuals were not sick people, 'for a perverse orientation is far from being a sickness'.[9] Furthermore, against the inclination of some of his most ardent followers, Freud maintained that homosexuality was no grounds to exclude trainee analysts.

A closer look at Freud's writing on homosexuality, however, reveals a more ambivalent legacy. The key to this ambivalence comes in Freud's con-ceptualisation of homosexuality as arrested development. This takes us back to Freud's schema of the acquisition of heterosexuality. Put very crudely, the Freudian infant is polymorphously perverse, a collection of drives that hardly differentiates between subject/object in the pursuit of release and satisfaction. In the process of becoming a subject, these drives are painfully civilised, culminating in the trials of the Oedipal complex, which for the male infant demands an acknowledgement of his father's sexual possession of his mother. The successful negotiation of this final stage of psychosexual development results in the acquisition of heterosexuality as the male, now an adult, goes in search of a heterosexual object to replace that earlier, painful repudiation. As commentators, not least feminists, have noted, the Freudian road to female heterosexuality lacked the clarity of male development, even as it was built more evidently on lack.

I have culled a very complex theory of sexuality and gender into a couple of lines. The more important point is that Freud stressed the radical contingency of sexual object choice. There was no innate heterosexuality, as such; it was a developmental achievement built upon the repudiation of polymorphous pleasures. We are all to some extent perverse, or would be if we could be. Homosexuality, in this model, was a station on the way to heterosexuality, not an illness or affliction of a particular breed of people. In fact Freud suggested that everyone was 'capable of making a homosexual object choice', and indeed had made one unconsciously.[10] However, the liberalism of this position could not disguise the idea that homosexuality remained arrested development—it was heterosexuality not yet fully realised. This did not mean that Freud believed adult homosexuals could be dragged into heterosexuality. As in most matters therapeutic, and unlike many of his successors, Freud was a pessimist on this point. A shift in adult sexual object choice was unlikely—nor was it necessary. Freud was careful not to confuse arrested development with psychopathology. Indeed, as Steven Frosh has pointed out, Freud made a clear theoretical distinction between disturbances of the sexual aim (perversions), and homosexuality in which there was a variation in object choice but not otherwise in the structure of sexuality (inversion).[11] One hundred years later, analysts are still tripping up on the distinction.

The liberalism of Freud's position, even with its limitations, was lost after his death. For the psychoanalytic world, homosexuality became associated with perversion and psychopathology. This reading of homosexuality drew on Freud's teleological model of psychosexual development while quietly dropping his unsettling theories on the variability of the sexual object. No longer a fragile achievement, heterosexuality became a prerequisite of individual maturity and mental health. Nowhere was this more evident than in the United States where analysts, from the inception of psychoanalysis, 'have tended to view homosexuality with disapproval and have actually wanted to get rid of it altogether'.[12] Abelove traces the moralism inherent in American psychoanalysis, especially evident in leading analytic figures like Sandor Rado, Irvng Beiber and Charles Socriades, all of whom argued passionately for homosexuality as perversion. These analysts, and many like them, effortlessly substituted Freud's descriptive theories of sexuality with a proscriptive heterosexuality. There were some notable exceptions. Heinz Kohut, for a time President of the American Psychoanalytic Association, not only saw homosexuality as simply one expression of narcissism (and not by definition an unhealthy choice) but also pondered the social conditions which deemed heterosexuality normative.[13] Kohut's views, however, were a minority. As a medical and cultural authority on human development, psychoanalysis reigned supreme during the 1940s and 1950s, and its treatment of homosexuals during this golden era was lamentable. The radical edge of Freudian theory was blunted in the United States, and in the postwar period American psychoanalysis ossified into a conservative and normalising force. Little wonder that feminists and gay activists would later nominate psychoanalysis as a bulwark against change.

Matters were hardly better in postwar Britain. Melanie Klein, a brilliant clinician and theoretician and immensely influential on the course of British psychoanalysis, viewed homosexuality as a flight from reality. Her theories, too, were complex, but she followed the developmental strand of Freudian theory in conceptualising homosexuality as a failure to negotiate success-fully the Oedipal conflicts. Klein, however, was more emphatic in stressing that homosexuality was a negative object choice.[14] In her clinical work Klein nominated heterosexuality as a major criterion for the termination of an analysis, along with 'capacity for love, object-relations and work, and certain characteristics of the ego which make up for mental stability'.[15] With her emphasis upon unconscious fantasy and her assumption that infants are born with an innate knowledge of complementary genital difference, Klein viewed homosexuality as originating from the paranoid-schizoid position. Adult homosexuals, from a strictly Kleinian perspective, can only manage part-object relations. They are 'driven by envious destructive phantasies arising from their failure to achieve the depressive position and the capacity for whole-object relations'.[16]

As late as 1990 Hanna Segal, a Kleinian psychoanalyst and training analyst with the British Institute of Psychoanalysis, could conclude that 'there is some reality sense and some innate idea about the parental couple and creative sexuality which is attacked by homosexuality'.[17] Again the message is clear. Homosexuality is a flight from reality, a sexuality devoid of creativity and mature relating. Elsewhere in the psychoanalytic world, ana-lysts such as Janine Chasseguet-Smirgel and Joyce McDougall have echoed the interpretation of homosexuality as a regressive flight from reality, attribu-table to either a systemic weakness in superego functioning or a desire to reinvent a more palatable primal scene.[18]

A certain *rapprochement* between psychoanalytic and homosexual cul-tures has occurred, with the American Psychoanalytic Association issuing a 1991 statement opposing discrimination in the admission of lesbians and gay men to training institutes, some eighteen years after the American Psy-chiatric Association deleted homosexuality from its *Diagnostic and Statistical Manual*.[19] With the rise in identity movements and the establishment of a gay and lesbian politics, it has been impossible for psychoanalytic institutions to insulate themselves completely from wider cultural change. Still, too often trainee therapists' homosexuality *per se* is deemed a disqualifying feature, even if this rejection is obscured in psychoanalytic niceties. And too often, of course, homosexual analysands find themselves in a position where their sexual choices—conscious and unconscious—are not given the same respect as their heterosexual counterparts. The terror of homosexuality runs deep in psychoanalysis. Whether they describe it as narcissistic, primitive and pre-Oedipal, a flight from reality, or an envious attack on the creativity of heterosexuality, psychoanalytic accounts of homosexuality can make for grim reading.

Psychologist Steven Frosh sheds a suggestive light on this terror. In reviewing what he describes as 'the incoherence of much of the psycho-analytic account of homosexuality', Frosh suggests that psychoanalytic institutions have used homosexuality as a means to cover their own conflicts around acceptance, creativity and sexuality. Psychoanalysis has trod a rocky road to social acceptance, and even today there are many commentators happy to declare the project dead. Psychoanalytic homophobia, Frosh reasons, has historically involved a grab by the profession for respectability and wider cultural legitimacy. He writes: 'It is as if the profession has said, unconsciously, "We may deal with all that is disturbing and disreputable in the human psyche, but at least we are normal: we hate homosexuals"'.[20] This could be expressed another way. In a profession immersed in ambivalence, psychoanalysis needs its certainties. Homosexuality as perversion has provided one such certainty, a marker against which the unruliness of sexual life might be ordered. In other words, psychoanalysis does not simply describe perversion, it regularly creates and cultivates it, as the debate from the Fortieth International Congress of Psychoanalysis showed. Put cheekily, there is something perverse in the psychoanalytic imagining of homosexuality, a part-object relationship if ever there was one.

Psychoanalysis and the history of homosexual critique

Against the odds, some social theorists of homosexuality have deployed psychoanalytic insights in the study of queer life. Dennis Altman, one of the earliest theorist of gay liberation, returned to Freud via Herbert Marcuse in his landmark 1971 text *Homosexual*. Altman drew upon Freud's concept of polymorphous perversity to argue for an innate human bisexuality. Civilisation, and late capitalism in particular, had forced men and women into surplus repression, denying their true sexual natures and creating the artificial social categories of heterosexual and homosexual. For Altman, the liberation of homosexuals was the first step in a wider reclaiming of an authentic sexuality, as humankind finally fulfilled its creative potential: 'If man- and womankind reaches the point where it is able to dispense with the categories of homo- and heterosexuality the gain will be well worth the loss'.[21] This was an unabashedly millenarian manifesto, at odds with the bleaker tone of Freudian metapsychology, but at least Altman saw a role for the unconscious in imagining new social arrangements. Thirty years later, his utopianism renounced, Altman could still find a place for Freud in social critique. In *Global Sex* Altman mounted the case for a psychoanalytic materialism to appreciate better the sexual dynamics of globalisation.

In the early days of gay liberation politics, Altman's optimistic reworking of Freud proved popular. In Australia gay liberationists enthusiastically welcomed the idea of an innate bisexuality, declaring that 'We are all gay, we are all straight'. This heady embrace was always more theoretical than practical, and when the promised polymorphously perverse revolution failed to materialise, references to a Freudian bisexuality quickly slipped away. By the mid-1970s the concept of a discrete homosexuality had prevailed. Politically the creation of a distinct gay identity made sense, for it provided the conceptual underpinning of identity politics and the gay community-building of the 1980s. The emergence of HIV/AIDS gave weight to this political imperative.[22] Psychoanalysis, however, was a victim of these shifts. The Freudo-Marxist tradition espoused by Altman was shelved in favour of another strand of gay theory and politics which saw psychoanalysis as 'the enemy incarnate', and not without some good cause.[23] This anti-psychoanalytic climate was especially acute in lesbian feminist circles, for whom psychoanalysis was the embodiment of sexism and homophobia. Kate Millet, an early and influential voice of 1970s feminism, described Freud as 'the strongest individual counter-revolutionary force in the ideology of sexual politics'.[24] Many lesbian feminists today would still happily agree with Millet's summation of Freud and the psychoanalytic project.

Psychoanalysis, then, provided a perfect punching bag for theorists of sexual identity, especially in the English-speaking world. It loomed as an immovable and reactionary force against which lesbians and gays could define their own liberated selves and progressive politics. And as we have seen, the psychoanalytic establishment provided fertile ground for such anti-psychoanalytic self-definition, not least in its sexual orthodoxies. Yet even as gay and lesbian theorists rejected the institutions and practice of psychoanalysis, many continued to speak a language indebted to psychoanalysis, albeit a bowdlerised form. Matters of the psyche did not go away, and questions of the self and the uncertain creation of identity continued to preoccupy many gays and lesbians. But without the benefit of psychoanalysis as 'a grammar of the emotions' this preoccupation regularly came up short.[25] Thus gay and lesbian life could invest much in the cultivation of 'gay pride', without considering adequately the denial of shame. And while the achievement of strong and vibrant social/political identities was celebrated, a consideration of the extent to which these sexual identities were idealised—and built partially upon a process of unconscious splitting and projection—was often neglected.[26]

Into the queer 1990s the conscious rejection of psychoanalysis in much homosexual critique took a sharper turn. This was most notable in the humanities, where the theoretical legacy of Michel Foucault was profound. According to Eli Zarestky, Foucault's discursive histories of sexuality rejected the distinction between inner and outer worlds, thus discarding the concept of internalisation which has so preoccupied psychoanalysis (although it should be noted there are widely divergent accounts of internalisation, depending upon one's psychoanalytic school). The idea of the individual was replaced with a new, Foucauldian conception of the subject, one which dismissed 'any conception of "instincts," drives, "inner world," "psychic reality," or the like'.[27] As I've noted, this shift to discourses and regimes of power was especially popular with historians and sociologists, for whom the idea of an inner world has always been troubling. Where, after all, was the evidence of an unconscious? In what archive, text or focus group? The leap of faith required to consider the psychoanalytic proved unpalatable for many queer historians and sociologists, and in Foucault they found the ideal theoretical justification not to try.

Christopher Lane, however, argues that the queer followers of Foucault have outstripped their master in rejecting psychoanalysis. Lane notes that Foucault did not include Freud in his critique of the repressive hypothesis, nor did he nominate pre-1940s psychoanalysis as a site of power/knowledge. It was the utopianism of the later Freudo-Marxists which Foucault rejected. In fact, Lane concludes, a more attentive reading of Foucault would show that 'Foucault represents psychoanalysis as an ally for lesbians and gay men precisely against narrow contemporaneous emphases on sexual norma-tivity'.[28] The fear, however, that any engagement with psychoanalysis will involve a trip down the royal road of desire to fixed identity categories, has meant few historians or sociologists have been willing to risk psychoanalyti-cally informed queer research of any hue. In the present moment of post-structuralism, an interest in looking beyond the gleam of discursive surfaces is too often deemed suspect.

The inner and outer world of queer perversion

Lest I overstate my case, I should note the calls for a *rapprochement* between gay/lesbian/queer social critique and psychoanalysis. A minority of voices has called for the deployment of psychoanalysis in studying homosexuality, although most of them have been British. More widely, such eminent theorists of sexuality and gender as Nancy Chodorow and Anthony Giddens have written psychoanalytically informed social research. A starting point for many of these writers has been a return to Freud's reflections on the variability of the erotic object. For Chodorow all sexualities are compromise formations—they are all to some degree neurotic, including your garden-variety heterosexuality.[29] There are, in other words, multiple outcomes to the Oedipal complex that may be deemed 'good enough', to poach a phrase from Winnicott. Giddens echoes this approach in his writing on 'plastic sexuality'. Whatever normal sexuality might be, he argues, it 'is simply one type of life style among others'.[30] Giddens also challenges the psychoanalytic world to rethink its investment in a typography of perversion. Confronting orthodox readings of the intra-psychic with the enormous social and cultural changes of recent decades, Giddens suggests that 'What used to be called perversions are merely ways in which sexuality can legitimately be expressed and self-identity defined'.[31]

Some critics might fear Giddens goes too far here, sacrificing the psycho-analytic for a contemporary cosmopolitanism. But he does return us to that problematic touchstone of psychoanalysis—perversion. By now we would expect that psychoanalytic and queer readings of perversion would differ radically. But by how much? To finish off, I want briefly to cite competing accounts of a contemporary 'perversion'—gay fist-fucking.

Fist-fucking, or 'fisting' as it is commonly called, is the delicate insertion of the hand into another's anus or vagina. While it is not an exclusively gay sexual practice, it is fair to say that in queer life fisting has been celebrated and codified. Recently queer theorists have picked up on this phenomenon. Anthropologist Gayle Rubin describes fisting as 'a truly original invention', and 'perhaps the only sexual practice invented in this [twentieth] century'. She notes how fisting became popular in the leather gay male community during the early 1970s, 'and then spawned its own unique sub-cultural elaboration and institutionalisation'.[32] While Rubin appreciates fisting from the perspective of community-building and identity creation, David Halperin takes a rigorously poststructuralist approach. Following Foucault, Halperin argues that 'the emergence of fist-fucking as both a sexual and sub-cultural phenomenon ... has the potential to contribute to redefining both the meaning and practice of sex'.[33] The argument here is that fisting shatters the familiar narrative of sexual desire by redistributing and remapping the body's erotic sites. More than that, these new pleasures have the potential to transform our understanding of the relationship between the self and sexuality, or more accurately, how the modern self is formed through a dis-course of sexuality. In Halperin's words, fisting 'disarticulates the psychic and bodily integration of the self to which a sexual identity has become attached'.[34]

Halperin's wish to disarticulate the psychic encapsulates a queer rejec-tion of psychoanalysis. Fisting, in this account, is a purely discursive oppor-tunity, not an intra-psychic event. Indeed, any register of perversion appears unsustainable in this post-Foucauldian turn. Not so for Larry O'Connell, a gay British psychoanalytic psychotherapist working with gay male clients. While anxious to reclaim the concept of the variability of the object, and highly critical of the psychoanalytic treatment of homosexuals, O'Carroll does not dismiss the perverse. This becomes clear in his discussion of 'Vince', a client who enjoyed fisting. O'Carroll interprets Vince's 'love' of fisting as the equation of intimacy with psychic catastrophe. Where Rubin describes fisting as 'seducing the jumpiest and tightest muscles in the body', O'Carroll emphasises how 'the anus is massively traumatised by the fist'.[35] In a transferential sense, O'Carroll views Vince's revelation late in therapy of his passion for fisting as an attempt to reduce his therapy to shit. Beyond the consulting room, O'Carroll decides that Vince's proclivities 'which sought to establish a hyper-real intimacy of invasion of his and other men's bodies, represented the reverse side of what he had been unable to experience in his life—sustaining, trustworthy intimacy'.[36]

The differences between this interpretation of fisting and the nonpsychoanalytic accounts of Rubin and Halperin are stark. O'Carroll finally defines fisting as belonging to the perverse sublime. In this reading, fisting is an attempt to deny the terror of intimacy by a triumph over the other. Drawing upon Klein's concept of manic defence, O'Connell argues that in using the object in the way it does, perversion seeks to annul the other, to obliterate the pain of psychic reality that comes with recognising the other's autonomy.[37] So while Rubin celebrates fisting as a basis for new communities, O'Carroll discovers a metaphor for the terror of intimacy. And although O'Carroll and Halperin share an interest in disintegration, their competing models of subjectivity produce very different versions of the same event. In fisting, O'Carroll finds the omnipotent annihilation of the other; Halperin a deeper ethical relationship with the self.

I'm not sure that we can reconcile these two interpretations. It would be unwise to expect a happy coupling of psychoanalysis and discourse theory. But I think we can use each to interrogate the other, to help map the complex, overlapping worlds of the intrapsychic, the intersubjective and the social. O'Carroll settles too easily for fisting as perversion. It is as if he too needs to find some psychoanalytic respectability, and discovering a sure-fire perversion is his means. Perhaps for Vince fisting is a flight from intimacy, but the analytic fit is a touch too tight for my liking. Other possible readings of fisting disappear in O'Carroll's consulting room—fisting can only represent the annihilation of the self and other, a disastrous collapse of the inner world. Alternatively, for Halperin fisting is the subversive play of surfaces, ironic in a sexual act that involves such depth. Questions of fantasy and intersubjectivity recede the more his discourse theory intrudes. Even Rubin's softer social constructionist approach shrugs off the unconscious. In the happy celebration of community-building, the power of individual emotion comes a poor second.

Imagine a third way if you will. While fisting may provide a new sociality, for some individuals it may also represent a flight from intimacy, a perversion if you like. Or it may not. Certainly O'Carroll overlooks recent psychoanalytic writing on sex that suggests 'a degree of depersonalisation ... may enhance the experience of both partners, and may heighten not only excitement but emotional contact'.[38] Nor does he consider those who believe fisting involves a spiritual experience, trust, intimacy, consideration and communication.[39] I believe these questions of fantasy and the inter-subjective remain crucial in the study of queer life, which is why I'm reluctant to relinquish the psychoanalytic. Yet psychoanalysis has its flaws, and historically the easy reliance on perversion has been one of them. To dispense with the perverse, however, is to deny the existence and possibility of individual pain, of addictions and relationships which drain the self, 'binding its creative energy into obsessions so private they are often unreadable to others'.[40]

We need both, then—psychoanalytic and non-psychoanalytic critique—to appreciate the inner and outer world of queer life. This takes us further down the path of uncertainty, to a world where relationships with ourselves and others are always a mix of the creative and the destructive.

5

Displacing Indigenous Australians: Freud's *Totem and Taboo*

Maggie Nolan

SIGMUND FREUD'S *Totem and Taboo* was originally published in four volumes over two years (1912–13) with the title *Some Points of Agreement Between the Mental Lives of Savages and Neurotics*. This marked the first convergence of the two newly emerging disciplines (and series of disciplinary procedures) that we now know of as anthropology and psychoanalysis. Freud reasoned in *Totem and Taboo* that 'a comparison between the psychology of primitive peoples, as it is taught by social anthropology, and the psychology of neurotics, as it has been revealed by psycho-analysis, will be bound to show numerous points of agreement and will throw new light upon familiar facts in both sciences'.[1] In this way, Freud attempts to undertake what amounts to a collective case study of 'the most backward and miserable of savages, the aborigines of Australia'.[2]

It is difficult not to respond to such a racist formulation with abhorrence. However, Freud's adherence to a racist economy based around the notion of the savage does not necessarily mean that psychoanalysis cannot provide us with any insights into such formulations. To remove the unconscious or psychic motivation from analysis because some theorisations of the unconscious have emerged within a racist epistemology would require the renewed assumption that the rational precepts of consciousness can and will explain everything. Yet is it possible to think adequately about colonial practices without indefinite concepts like fantasy and desire, projection and displacement? Is it possible, moreover, to challenge colonialism and its contemporary effects without putting into question the status of the subject?

So, somewhat problematically, I hope to retain psychoanalysis as a set of conceptual tools to think about colonialism, and simultaneously consider it a part of that armoury of legitimating knowledges that helps to comprise the colonial project. Following the lead of Gilles Deleuze and Felix Guattari, I refuse 'to play "take it or leave it"' with psychoanalysis.[3]

Psychoanalysis, like all sciences, disciplines and epistemologies, emerged out of a certain set of historical circumstances. Freud, moreover, was not merely a product of his time, but a brilliant analyst of it; and psychoanalysis, for all its situatedness, is an important contribution to understanding the psychic world of the colonising Western subject and its effects. My argument follows Deleuze and Guattari's reading of Freudian psychoanalysis to the extent that it works with the assumptions that desire is contingent, variable and polymorphous, that it does not have a specific aim and object, and that it is not localised in the operation of the genitals. Deleuze and Guattari's reading of Freud suggests that the Oedipus complex was a radical insight, the implications of which Freud refused to acknowledge. In so doing, his insight about the socialisation of desire was repressed, and the Oedipus complex and its resolution were made fundamental to so-called normal development, making the patriarchal nuclear family a universal and necessary form within traditional psychoanalysis. My narrative attempts to historicise psychoanalytic theory in order to think about the Oedipal structuring of desire that Freud identified and analysed as a socio-historical effect that characterises the capitalist and colonialist social formation.

The most subversive contribution of psychoanalysis is arguably its theorisation of human subjectivity, which interrogates and decentres the individual's pretensions to self-knowledge and the concomitant claims to represent reason and reality. This presents a paradox: psychoanalysis staked out its epistemological claim in the realm of unknowability—the unconscious—a realm that, according to Freud, can only leave traces of its existence. While displacing the self-mastery of the subject, Freud maintains a teleological belief in the progress of human reason and the all-encompassing possibilities of science. 'The deficiencies in our description would probably vanish', Freud asserts, 'if we were already in a position to replace the psychological terms by physiological or chemical ones . . . Biology is truly a land of unlimited possibilities'.[4]

Freud's faith in science, however, is always haunted by his own proposition that the subject is inevitably inhabited by an unknowable otherness. Psychoanalysis, then, is complicated by more than just the constitutive instabilities that inhabit any form of discourse; it inevitably disrupts its own premises, and my reflections on *Totem and Taboo* seek to work with this disruptive potentiality.

On the opening page of *Totem and Taboo*, Freud argues that the 'savage' is, in a certain sense, 'our' contemporary:

> There are men still living who, as we believe, *stand very near to* primitive man, far nearer than we do, and whom we therefore regard as his direct heirs and *representatives*. Such is our view of those whom we describe as savages or half-savages; and their mental life must have a peculiar interest for us if we are right in *seeing it* as *a well-preserved picture* of an early stage of our own development [emphasis added].[5]

For Freud, the 'primitive man' he is seeking to analyse can only be perceived hauntingly through a complex series of relationships to Indigenous Australians who are made to stand near to, in for (represent), and be a well-preserved image of the savagery of Europe's prior selves. In other words, 'primitive man', the subject under discussion, is not quite there at all.

The absence of the savage was not a phenomenon unique to Freud, nor was it particularly new. Phantasmatic descriptions of the savage inhabitants of places outside Europe had been circulating in Europe before Europeans had even seen those inhabitants.[6] Unsurprisingly, early theorisations of the savage, Jean-Jacques Rousseau's 'noble savage' in the 'Discourse on Inequality' for example, are deeply contradictory. Not only did the savage represent a state of freedom in nature, so-called savage societies were simultaneously conceived as structured around a system of authoritarian patriarchal lineages. Yet Rousseau and many of his contemporaries considered a society just and free in so far as it minimised the extent to which one's father's position determined one's own, a challenge to patriarchal authority that was characteristic of the debates within emergent enlightenment thought.

These debates relied upon conjectural histories of the formation of civil society, that is, civilisation—a term that came into general use towards the end of the eighteenth century, and was explicitly linked to the idea of human progress and its cumulative achievements. The contract theorists who fuelled these debates, of whom Rousseau is a prime example, argued that a new form of political right is created through a contract, freely entered into, that replaces patriarchal rule. In the story of the social contract, the father is superseded by the sons who transform the father's patriarchal right into civil government.

Carole Pateman has drawn out some of the gender implications of these narratives and how they naturalise a sexual contract where men's freedom rests on women's subjection.[7] Contractual society, rather than opposing or superseding patriarchy, is the means through which modern fraternal patriarchy, which structures contemporary civil society, is constituted.

Such a manoeuvre was enabled because conjectural histories relied on a human nature that originated in the primordial past. So I would like to propose an alternative narrative that interprets these debates through the lens of more recent intersecting socio-political transformations in Europe that might be thought of as constituting the conditions for the production of a historically situated Oedipus complex.

Philip Barker argues that in north-west Europe, 'perhaps up until the tenth century, there was no single system of inheritance and social identification; on the contrary, the situation was one of wide diversity, from those suggestive of maternal descent, to those of exclusively paternal descent'.[8] However, from about the tenth century there were two significant changes: 'first the end of partability for patrimonial lands, and secondly, the uniform preference for inheritance along the male line only'.[9] As Barker notes, under a system of primogeniture, inheritance became the central locus of disputes between fathers and sons: 'There is nothing unconscious about this rebellion: to kill the father is an integral part of claiming an inheritance speedily from the moment of coming of age'.[10]

Barker elucidates the range of strategies that were used to support these changes: 'strengthening the indissolubility of marriage, dissuading from concubinage, and encouraging the production of legitimate heirs from one socially sanctioned conjugal unit'.[11] The church intervened to support these aims through the legitimisation and regulation of relationships, which led to the widespread restructuring of the family towards a patriarchal nuclear family as the dominant economic unit. This resulted in the structuring and monitoring of sexual relations, and a concomitant anxiety about sexual pleasure that may have contributed to the institution of private confession as the annual practice of all Christians after the fourth Lateran Council of 1215. In this way, a dialogue with the self, which focused specifically on the question of sexual desire, was created.

Accompanying these political changes in medieval Europe was the increasing interiorisation of alphabetic literacy, a technology that, with the institution of confession, played a significant part in the transformation of consciousness that is associated with the modern age. As Walter Ong points out, the interiorisation of self-reflexive modes of consciousness enabled by literacy is 'a particularly pre-emptive and imperialist activity that tends to assimilate other things to itself'.[12] Ong argues that alphabetic literacy facilitates categorical thought, sequential thinking and a far greater concern with the past and the future. If this is so, then encounters with radically different cultures from the medieval period onwards could be readily understood in temporally progressive classificatory terms, out of which both racial theory and evolutionary anthropology may well have emerged.

By the time debates about the nature of contractual civil society emerged in the late seventeenth century, these transformations were well established. Emerging print technology allowed for the reproducibility and widespread circulation and dissemination of both ideas and modes of consciousness. The regulation of sexuality continued to be central to these debates. The increasing faith in reason, as enabling social progress, was accompanied by a concomitant anxiety about sexuality, particularly women's sexuality. Sexuality, then, came to be seen as the antithesis of reason, because it destabilised the surety of legitimate inheritance, thereby jeopardising the very terms of civil society. Women, considered unable to participate in the modes of reason and rationality that underpin the social contract, were thereby consigned to what we now think of as the domestic sphere, leading to the pseudo-separation of the political and the domestic spheres. This separation continues, to some extent, to characterise contractual, or what we might now think of as capitalist, social relations.

These changes had a number of significant effects, both on the structure of the family and the individual. They enabled the production and stabilisation of secure and self-reflexive identities through a structure of patrilineal heritage. At the same time, the concerns of reproduction and child-rearing were increasingly separated from the public domain which led to the narrow and restricted identifications that are characteristic of the Oedipalised subject.

These changes necessarily impacted upon the production of knowledge, one outcome being the emergence of the discipline of anthropology at the end of the nineteenth century. The conditions that I have argued might have constituted an Oedipus complex are the same conditions that produced the study of anthropology and, necessarily, the knowledge it produced. Henrika Kuklick argues that the emergence of anthropology was, in part, an effect of the widespread concern with the issue of inheritance which, as we have seen, was central to contractual civil society and the ideology of meritocracy: 'the belief that an individual's wealth, status and power should reflect the worth of their achievements rather than the social standing of their parents'.[13] Anthropology was thus concerned with the question of the status of the modern individual and structuring the relationship to the authority of the father, and inheritances from him, within a biologistic framework. Not only did anthropology emerge out of questions concerning inheritance, it made questions of inheritance—the development of law, the family, private property and the state—its object of study.

E. B. Tylor, the first professor of anthropology in Britain, and considered the 'father' of anthropology, published *Researches into the Early History of*

Mankind and the Development of Civilization in 1865. It was, according to George Stocking, 'a methodological exercise—an attempt to see how far a study of cultural similarities might carry one toward reconstructing the actual early history of mankind'.[14] With the publication of Charles Darwin's *The Descent of Man* in the same year as *Primitive Culture*, anthropologists increasingly came to apply biological evolutionary theory to the socio-cultural sphere. In 1865 another British anthropologist, John Ferguson McLennan, had published *Primitive Marriage* which illustrates the contemporary concern with human, and particularly female, sexual desire. For McLennan, marriage was an institution that enabled 'certainty of male parentage' through 'the appropriation of women to particular men' and the 'conception of conjugal fidelity'.[15] The evolution upward from promiscuity and polyandry was the evolution towards the culmination of civilisation in the mid-Victorian patriarchal nuclear family, and the monogamous sexual propriety that governed it.

McLennan, through his interest in 'primitive marriage', linked animism and exogamy, a term he coined to refer to marriage outside the group, through the idea of totemism in 'The Worship of Animals and Plants', written in 1869–70. He took Tylor's animistic thesis and added a sociological dimension. McLennan defined totemism as the appropriation of a special fetish to a tribe. According to McLennan, tribes in the totem stage believed themselves to be descended from some animal or plant that was their 'symbol or emblem' and 'religiously regarded' or 'taboo', recognised kinship through the mother, and followed 'exogamy as their marriage law'.[16] McLennan's ideas on both primitive marriage and totemism proved to be extremely influential for Freud.

Likewise was Sir James Frazer's entry on 'Totemism' (1885) for the T volume of *Encyclopaedia Britannica*. This three-page entry turned into a thirteen-volume book, an illustration of Frazer's all-consuming methodology which is exemplary of the epistemological all-inclusiveness that characterised the Western faith in the accumulation of knowledge. Frazer's Tylorian approach, which assumed that the socio-cultural sphere is governed by laws that science can discover through the use of empirical reasoning, 'sifted the arguments in every branch of the new discipline and asserted an orthodoxy'.[17]

By the last decade of the nineteenth century, almost all anthropologists agreed that most primitive societies were structured around kinship relations, organised on the basis of descent groups that were exogamous and related by a series of exchange marriages. Most also adhered to McLennan's Doctrine of Survivals which was based on Lewis Henry Morgan's classificatory system. This doctrine asserted that, like extinct species, primeval institutions are preserved in fossil form in contemporary ceremonies and kinship terminologies of so-called primitive peoples and these bear witness to long-dead practices. This belief was maintained in spite of the fact that in an Australian anthropological expedition undertaken by Lorimer Fison and Alfred Howitt in the 1870s, Fison had to admit that kinship terminologies were no simple matter and that 'after years of inquiry into this matter, the humiliating confession must be made that I am hopelessly puzzled'.[18]

It was from these epistemological domains that Freud, in *Totem and Taboo*, assembled his own psychoanalytic interpretations of the models of anthropology. Freud's argument, which extends Darwin's hypothesis of the primal horde, culminates in the positing of a primal horde dominated by a powerful father who possessed all the available women. In an event that Freud claims 'might be described as historical', the sons, in their rage and frustration, joined together, killed the father, and then cannibalised him.[19] Because of the ambivalent structure of the instincts, however, the brothers felt both love and hate for their father, encouraging guilt and remorse in the post-parricide world. They therefore set him up as a totem, and incorporated his terror within them. Thus, as with the development of the individual's superego, what had been an external authority became incorporated internally as legislative guilt. This is the Oedipal moment, a moment that both others the self and marks the beginnings of civilisation through a fraternal pact.

Although Freud asserts that it 'goes without saying' that the 'cannibal savages of the primal horde ... devoured their victim as well as killing him',[20] he reiterates its centrality a number of times, and goes so far as to invoke the spectacle of that first totem meal. Freud makes the motive of such cannibalisation transparent: 'in the act of devouring him they accomplished their identification with him, and each one of them acquired a portion of his strength'.[21] As Mikkel Borch-Jacobsen suggests, 'What is at stake in this struggle is now quite clear: the acquisition of an identity. Desire culminates in a murder and a cannibalistic sacrificial meal because it is directed towards the acquisition of an identity by means of the assimilation of the other.'[22] According to Freud, the guilty memory of the murder of the primal father has 'left ineradicable traces in the history of humanity'.[23] These 'ineradicable traces' that continue to haunt humanity, who become bearers of this transmitted and inherited act, exist only residually and indeterminately in relation to the subject. For Freud then, the process of identification, through which individual identity is acquired, will always necessarily be Oedipal.

The hypothesis of the primal horde provides Freud with a historical grounding for the Oedipus complex, a touchstone of orthodoxy in psychoanalytic thought. By positing an actual historical event, the primal horde narrative answers the question of how the specifically Oedipal ordering of desire comes about. Without the primal horde, there is no Oedipus complex. Freud claims to be committed to historical process. He says, for example, in relation to the question of taboo: 'I hope to be able . . . to make it probable that a definite historical chain of events is concealed behind the fate of this concept'.[24] Yet the Oedipus complex is not the effect of such a process; it instigates it. In this way, Freud banishes the history that produced the Oedipal subject.

Freud's commitment to the historical progress of evolutionary anthropology, moreover, situates the Indigenous Australians who were under investigation as temporally prior to the Europeans investigating them. This is most evident in his discussions of the realm of sexual desire where the Aboriginal Australian is assumed to be more aligned with the primitive forces of the id than with the rational ego:

> it is enough to draw attention to the great care which is devoted by the Australians . . . to the prevention of incest. It must be admitted that these savages are even more sensitive on the subject of incest than we are. They are probably liable to a greater temptation to it and for that reason stand in need of fuller protection.[25]

This situating of Indigenous Australians in another time, or 'allochronism' as Johannes Fabian has named it, is even more explicit in a later section of *Totem and Taboo*: 'It is therefore of no small importance that we are able to show that these same incestuous wishes, which are later destined to become unconscious, are still regarded by savage peoples as immediate perils against which the most severe measures of defence must be enforced'.[26]

So in Freud's narrative, the modern Western subject is conceived of as the effect of the unfolding of history from an originary point, a point to which Indigenous Australians are temporally more proximate. Contemporary Indigenous Australians thus became objects of study for what they could tell investigators about the prehistory of the investigators themselves. Rather than thinking about Aboriginal societies as differently evolved, or colonial contact as an encounter with alterity, Indigenous peoples were incorporated into a European narrative of identity (in much the same way as the primal sons incorporated the father) that enabled and justified their supersession. This manoeuvre turns the narrative of the Oedipus complex into the narrative of the colonisation and assimilation of the colonial other.

The primal horde hypothesis, a phantasmatic extension and effect of the historically situated Oedipus complex, returns to the origin in order to understand, control and validate the present. This return allows for the universalisation of the Oedipus complex. Freud's hypothesis cannot admit the possibility of non-Oedipalised subjects, or the possibility of other types of familial or socio-cultural arrangements, or even the possibility that socio-sexual desire might be organised in a range of diverse ways. For Freud, the Oedipus complex is necessarily centred around the patriarchal nuclear family, a family that is subsequently both naturalised and dehistoricised.

In *Totem and Taboo* Freud draws on the 'recorded facts' of anthropology for his authority, and submits them to analysis 'as though they formed part of the symptoms presented by a neurosis'.[27] The recorded facts that Freud refers to, however, emerged out of anthropological knowledge, a form of knowledge that I have argued is itself an effect of processes of Oedipalis-ation. As Deleuze and Guattari assert: 'We never dreamed of saying that psychoanalysis invented Oedipus. Everything points in the opposite direc-tion: the subjects of psychoanalysis arrive already Oedipalized.'[28]

Perhaps it is possible to think about the recorded facts more sympto-matically. Freud suggests as much when he calls into question the entire project of *Totem and Taboo*, and the status of the recorded facts, in a footnote on the second page:

> Not only, however, is the *theory* of totemism a matter of dispute; the facts them-selves are scarcely capable of being expressed in general terms ... There is scarcely a statement that does not call for exceptions and contradictions. But it must not be forgotten that even the most primitive and conservative races are in some sense *ancient* races and *have a long past history behind them* during which their original conditions of life have been subject to much development and *distortion*. So it comes about that in those races in which totemism exists to-day, we may find it in various stages of decay and disintegration or in the process of transition to other social and religious institutions, or again in a stationary con-dition which may differ greatly from the original one. The difficulty in this last case is to decide whether we should regard the present state of things as a *true picture* of the significant features of the past or as a *secondary distortion* of them [emphasis added].[29]

This is the kind of detail that psychoanalysis cannot ignore. This footnote, literally a textual parapraxis, suggests that the anthropological texts that Freud himself cites might be characterised by the form of thinking peculiar to dreams and neuroses. Freud is suggesting that we cannot know whether the content of anthropological texts provides a 'true picture' of the ancient past, or whether, like the manifest content of dreams, it is the effect of series of distortions complete with a secondary revision, the purpose of which is 'to get rid of the disconnectedness and unintelligibility produced by the dream-work and replace it with a new meaning'. 'But this new meaning', Freud warns, is no longer the meaning of the dream-thoughts ... There is an intellectual function in us which demands unity, connection and intelligibility from and material, whether of perception or thought, that comes within its grasp; and if, as a result of special circumstances, it is unable to establish a true connection, it does not hesitate to fabricate a false one.[30]

In *Totem and Taboo*, Freud claims that he has arrived at the point of regarding a child's ambivalent relation to his parents, 'dominated as it is by incestuous longings, as the nuclear complex of neurosis', a complex to which, he states, 'we have given the name of "Oedipus complex"'.[31] In the same text, he also claims that the child 'finds relief from the conflict arising out of this double-sided, this ambivalent emotional attitude towards the father by displacing his hostile and fearful feelings on a *substitute* of his father'.[32] The mechanism of displacement is, according to Freud, difficult to recognise and contain: 'The instinctual desire is constantly shifting in order to escape the *impasse* and endeavours to find substitutes—substitute objects and substitute acts—in place of the prohibited ones'.[33] Is it possible to think about the practice of anthropology as one such substitutive act?

Perhaps we can think about the representations of Indigenous Australians as evolutionary forefathers that Freud uses and adheres to in *Totem and Taboo* as one of the sites of displacement for the modern, Western Oedipal subject. Freud's use in his footnote of the word 'distortion' (*entstellung*) to refer to the nature of the content of anthropological texts is significant, and he reminds us elsewhere that he uses it with 'the double meaning to which it has a claim but of which today it makes no use. It should mean not only "to change the appearance of something" but also "to put in another place, to displace"'.[34] This second, spatial or territorial meaning of distortion has particular resonances in the context of colonisation where this neurotic displacement is literally enacted.

It is significant, when considered from this perspective, that Freud would repeatedly use metaphors of colonisation and domination to describe the resolution of the Oedipus complex as the foundation for the control of desire: 'Civilization ... obtains mastery over the individual's dangerous desire for aggression by weakening and disarming it and by setting up an agency within him to watch over it, like a garrison in a conquered city'.[35] Similarly, in 'The Dissection of the Psychical Personality', Freud refers to the repressed as 'foreign territory' and the purpose of psychoanalytic therapy 'to strengthen the ego, to make it more independent of the superego, to widen its field of perception and enlarge its organisation, so that it can appropriate fresh portions of the id. Where id was, there ego shall be'.[36] That civilisation is associated with the ego and sexuality with the id, in an imperial relation, is clear in Freud's assertion that civilisation 'behaves towards sexuality as a people or a stratum of its population does which has subjected another one to its exploitation'.[37] Civilisation, here anthropomorphised, seeks to protect itself from aggression, yet it seems that it is only through aggression that such protection can be ensured. In these metaphors, it is difficult to say if the feared locus of aggression is the conquered or the conqueror.

Freud claims that the 'influences of civilization cause an ever-increasing transformation of egoistic trends into altruistic and social ones by an admixture of erotic elements'.[38] For Freud, barbaric acts are always attributable to archaic traces: 'It must be granted that all the impulses that society condemns as evil—let us take as representative the selfish and cruel ones—are of this primitive kind'.[39] It is the primitive within us, the forces at work in the id, Freud argues, that we need to guard against.

In this essay, I have proposed an alternative narrative of the Oedipus complex to the one that Freud presents in *Totem and Taboo*, one that attempts to think differently about the convergence of the Oedipal moment and the modern imperial period. My own conjectural history attempts to activate the disruptive potential of psychoanalysis to suggest that colonisation, rather than being the harbinger of civilisation, can be thought of as the enactment of violent fantasies of supersession and domination that are peculiar to the colonial psyche and its history. Anthropology and psychoanalysis, and the savage they posit, can from this perspective be seen as neurotic symptoms of the barbarity of colonisation that they seek to legitimise and displace.

II

Biography and identities

6

The tasks of political biography[1]

Judith Brett

To ADMIT TO USING psychoanalytic ideas in biographical work is immediately to find oneself on the defensive, facing a salvo of arguments ranging from 'Freud is bunk' to 'you cannot psychoanalyse the dead'. And as one argument is rebutted, a new one is produced, and then another, until the first one reappears in a slightly altered form: the language is so ugly; psychoanalysis is reductionist, determinist, anti-humanist, patriarchal; literature is a better guide to the inner life and, in these post-universalist days, Freud is of only historic interest. This essay is a defence of the role of psychoanalysis in political biography.

The task of political biography is to tell the story of a political life in such a way as to make that life intelligible. In describing this task, I am deliberately avoiding the word 'psychobiography', not only because there have been some very bad books published under this description, but also because I want to avoid its implication of the primacy of psychoanalytic ideas and concepts among the biographer's tools. Instead I want to advance a more modest claim, that psychoanalytic concepts and methods should be present in the biographer's tool kit. This does necessarily involve tackling some of the arguments against the applications of psychoanalysis to historical material, although I will not cover them all and recommend to interested readers Peter Gay's lucid little book *Freud for Historians* which deals in a systematic way with the most common arguments against the applications of psychoanalysis to history.

Leon Edel argues that contemporary biographies that do not use the knowledge of psychoanalysis are incomplete, belonging to a time when lives were entirely exterior and neglected the reflective and inner sides of human beings.[2] Few contemporary biographers are content to see themselves as chroniclers of the exterior life. They want also to convey something of what their subject thought and felt about the key events and conflicts and the passing moments of their life; to bring out something of their personality—the characteristic patterning of gestures and response which are uniquely theirs, the characteristic strategies which contribute to their successes and failures; and to convey something of the way they changed during the course of their life. The contemporary biographer moves continually between the outer and the inner, between the events and the culture of the times and the idiosyncratic and personally felt responses of the life.

Edel is writing from the experience of literary biography, where the biographer's subject, by definition, is a person who spends their life cultivating and transforming their inner life into words that others, including the biographer, can read. But what if you are writing about someone who themselves neglected their inner and reflective side, who lived in the external world of action and event, and who left little if any of the sorts of writing which seem to give some access to the inner life—no records of dreams, no diary entries about emotions, no intimate letters?

One solution is to look to the details of the private life. As Eric Erikson says, in psychoanalysis 'deeper' often seems to mean sexual and repressed.[3] Psychoanalysis can seem to be mainly useful to the biographer for its attention to what is hidden, taking place behind closed doors, in the innermost recesses of the private life. Psychoanalysis can thus seem a method particularly designed for digging up dirty secrets. It is this conception of psychoanalysis that evokes so much hostility as it seems concerned with the denigration and trivialisation of worthy public lives. This criticism aside, the problem with this conception of psychoanalysis is that it confines it to the investigation of the private life, and the private lives of some individuals may not be particularly illuminating. In an article on political biography, Kenneth Morgan writes, 'The relentless emphasis on Lloyd George's sexual adventures—real or alleged—for example can lead to extreme misinterpretation of the career of one who was above all, night and day, a supremely committed politician, obsessed with the issues of the time. Nothing, not even sex, could interfere with that'.[4]

The reliance of much psychoanalytic thinking on metaphors of depth maps easily onto a distinction between the public and the private life in which the private life seems to hold the clues to the meaning of the public life. Such a mapping though is misleading for the biographers of many politicians who are faced not only with a paucity of material, but with a private life that is scarcely lived. If psychoanalysis is to be useful to the political biographer, it must be useful in understanding the public life; and it must begin not with what is hidden and secret but with what is right in front of its nose—the publicness of the public life. It is, if you like, the publicness of the life that marks it as political. It is thus not so much a matter of searching for the real person behind the public person, but of realising that the public person is the real person and so learning to read the public political life for what it reveals about the distinctiveness of the person.

It has been argued that men who seek and win public political power share certain characteristics. Harold Lasswell, one of the first to apply Freud's ideas to the systematic study of political lives, argued that men who devote their lives to the pursuit of high public office seek power and deference in order to overcome estimates of the self which they regard as inappropriately low. Such men typically come from backgrounds which put them at some distance from the centres of power and significance in their society: colonials, small-town boys, members of minorities, those from the wrong side of the tracks or the blanket. Lasswell's theory aims to illuminate the lives not of those born to power, but of those who strive for it.[5]

Central to the psychology of such men, argues Lasswell, is the psychological mechanism of projection, by which inner conflicts are displaced onto objects in the outside world and dealt with there, generally rationalised in terms of the public interest. These men are externalisers, dealing with their inner conflicts and struggles not by changing themselves, but by changing, or attempting to change, the world. Fighting for the nation against colonial oppressors, serving the king, advancing the interests of a class or party—such men are also advancing their own interests, attempting to forge a pact between their own claims to power and deference and the interests of those they would represent. In popularly based politics ambition must be hitched to group goals, for it is only by successfully advancing such goals that the political type has any chance of reaching high office.

The close link between political ambition and self-interest is widely recognised in a settler democracy like Australia, where cynicism about politicians' motives has always been high. In the absence of a traditional governing class, Australian politics seems full of what Michael Kirby, arguing for a constitutional monarchy which would keep at least one job beyond their grasp, has called 'the pushing, shoving types'.[6] But while Lasswell's argument about the necessary link between projection and political ambition might lend support to this sort of real-world cynicism, it is also an argument about the deep sources of political energy, about what it is that makes some men and women go on fighting when others have compromised or called it a day and gone on to do other things with their lives. It is about what it is that makes some men and women unable to leave politics alone. One thinks of Maggie Thatcher and Bob Hawke. Here it is important to go beyond the easy cynicism which recognises the ambitious politician's pact between self-interest and general interest, and to see that great good may flow from such pacts, that the interest of the class or the nation may indeed be advanced by an ambitious man or woman seeking power and deference. Indeed Erik Erikson in *Young Man Luther* argues that in raising their deep personal conflicts to a general level such people may be catalysts for major social change.

Lasswell's work makes two major contributions to political biography: it points to the centrality of psychoanalytic theories about the self (theories of narcissism) for understanding political leaders, and in the mechanism of projection it gives the biographer a powerful tool for linking the inner life of their subject with the public life of the times. Both of these contributions challenge two of the most popular misconceptions about the limitations of psychoanalysis for biography: the first is that it is all about sex, and the second is that it is only interested in the individual and so is blind to history.

Is psychoanalysis all about sex?

In the view that psychoanalysis is all about sex, psychoanalysis becomes synonymous with the early work of Freud on the drives and his discovery of childhood sexuality. It thus seems to be about digging up dirty secrets, or reducing adult achievements to the playing out of childhood wishes. These misconceptions very easily slide into another one: that psychoanalysis is about pathology, and hence to apply it to so-called normal people is inappropriate.[7] Not only are these wrongheaded understandings of the complexity and contribution of Freud's work, but they completely ignore the development of psychoanalytic theory since Freud. It is not sufficient when dismissing psychoanalytically informed biography simply to make a few insulting remarks about Freud; one must also take account of the work of theorists since Freud. Of particular relevance to the essays in this collection is the work of Melanie Klein and the British Object Relations School, in particular Wilfred Bion and Donald Winnicott, as well as of the Americans Karen Horney and Heinz Kohut.

Despite their many differences, these psychoanalytic thinkers share a focus on understanding the way the human self emerges from the child's very early relations with its parents and develops through childhood and youth and into adult life. The experiences of childhood sexuality are thus placed in the context of the way in which the parents respond to the child's emerging self. From this perspective the core of the Oedipal crisis is not the sexual wish and its denial but a lesson about the limits and possibilities of the self. For the biographer, childhood experiences of humiliation may be far more important for understanding the adult subject than childhood sexual fantasies.

The argument here is not that sex is never of any relevance to the political biographer, but that psychoanalysis is about much more than the origins and vicissitudes of adult sexuality. In relation to some political lives, the biographer may indeed need to think a good deal about the subject's sexuality, particularly in political contexts where the subject's sexuality becomes part of the way in which they express their political power. One thinks here of the recent biography of Mao Zedong, or of the Ceausescus, or, more benignly, of Soekarno.

To a very great extent, liberal societies with their separation between the private individual and the authority of the public office keeps a check on the more florid aspects of human sexuality being brought in to play in the actual exercise of state power. Sadists, for example, do not get their hands on state power. But even in liberal democracies, the projection of a certain sexual style may be part of a politician's bid for public power; one thinks here of Jeff Kennett's flamboyant virility which is displayed as a sign of tough-minded worldliness and general lack of sentimentality.

Ambition and ideals

In his early foray into the field Lasswell stressed the ambitious politician's craving for deference, thereby putting too much weight on grievance as a source of energy for political lives. Grievance is undoubtedly a powerful source in many cases, but a more flexible theory of the self is needed by biographers dealing with a wide range of political lives. Some political biographers have found Karen Horney's work useful, in particular her *Neurosis and Human Growth: The Struggle Toward Self-realisation*, in which she develops the concept of an idealised self as a response to the insecurities and anxieties engendered by unempathic parenting.[8] Horney's discussion of the various forms of the construction and defence of an idealised self—the different paths taken by those who compulsively search for glory—is very suggestive for political biographers. Her formulation of the idealised self in terms of neurosis does, however, imply that the vicissitudes of self-realisation she describes are pathological.

The work of Heinz Kohut sharply breaks with this implication. Rather than seeing narcissism as a stage through which individuals pass in their development towards psychological maturity, Kohut argues that the construction and defence of the self's cohesion is a life-long task. Psychoanalysts thus need to rethink their generally negative evaluation of narcissism which is as implicated in the joys and creativity of human life as in its selfishness and destructiveness. His work pertains to all people, but it is especially helpful for political biographers who are often dealing with people extraordinarily endowed with self-regard.

Kohut looks in detail at the processes by which the idealised self is constructed, and he distinguishes two stages in this process. The first is the grandiose self of the very young child, who feels themself the centre of the universe and delights in their own existence. The second is the idealised self of the slightly older child who is starting to be aware of the relative powerlessness of children, but retains the sense of their own power and uniqueness through identification with an admired parent. 'I am perfect' becomes 'you are perfect but I am part of you, so I am still perfect'.[9] The grandiose self, Kohut argues, is the seat of ambition, the drive to reach the social position where one's true self will be recognised. The idealised self is seat of the self's desire to live up to and serve ideals. One is driven by ambition, but strives for one's ideals.[10] Throughout life there is an interaction between these two aspects of the self: one is driven by ambition to reach one's 'rightful' place, to receive one's due rewards and recognition, but one strives for one's ideals, to put one's life and talents at the service of something beyond the self, but with which the self is deeply identified.

Both ambition and ideals are of central interest to political biographers, and Kohut's work is very helpful in providing a dynamic model for thinking about the way these interact in a political life. Kohut leads one to ponder how and why one's subject invests a part of him or herself in political causes, ideas or institutions, and he is a check against the too easy cynicism of those who only see the self-serving ambition and fail to see as well the struggle to harness that ambition for some more general purpose.

In my thinking about Menzies, Kohut's formulation of the self as both driven by ambition and led by ideals was extremely helpful. Menzies was a man of powerful ambition who carried into adult life a pleasure in his own capacities and achievements that many of his contemporaries found extremely galling. But Menzies the man of ambition was not the whole story, despite what many of his critics would like to believe, for Menzies was determined to turn his ambition to good use, and strove to serve and protect loved ideals such as the British Empire, the law and parliamentary democracy. These ideals controlled and gave meaning to his ambition, although at times the tables turned and the ideals became transparent rationalisations for the ambition. Although it took me longer to see Menzies' commitment to his ideals than it did to see his driving ambition, when I did it gave me a more complex way of understanding his political life; and it gave me a basis for understanding the tenacity with which he hung onto his early ideals even when, as with the British Empire, their star had faded.[10]

The historical context

The second misconception implicitly challenged by Lasswell is that psycho-analysis is of little use to the central biographical task of making subjects intelligible in their historical context. This misconception derives from the view of psychoanalysis as primarily concerned with analysing individuals in terms of the working-out of ahistorical drives. From the beginning, however, psychoanalysis has been concerned with the traffic between the inner and the outer world, with how real experiences of the outer world are trans-formed by fantasy and the unconscious, and with how the objects of the outer world come to carry meanings derived from the inner world, through the processes of introjection and projection respectively. This is most developed in the work of Melanie Klein and the British Object Relations School.

Through introjection and projection one takes into or expels from the self thoughts, emotions and ideas. In introjection one makes part of the outer world one's own; in projection one disowns part of one's self and expels it into the outer world. These are the processes through which the institutions, people and events of the subject's life come to carry their emo-tions and fantasies, and so provide the biographer with ways of thinking about how the inner life of the subject is knitted together with the outer life of the times. Conventional life and times biography, by comparison, has few ways of showing the dynamic connections between the life and the times, except for notions such as influence which are far too weak to explain the passionate commitments and hatreds of political lives. There is thus much reliance on good descriptive writing to evoke the historical context, as well as frequent resort to truisms like 'in his love of England Menzies was a man of his times', which say nothing at all about the reasons for the particular intensity, even for his times, of Menzies' love of England.

Of course, in some aspects of a subject's life they may simply be of their times. As Freud said, 'sometimes a cigar is just a cigar'. There is no estab-lished way of determining when one's subject is revealing a part of their inner self rather than simply behaving according to the accepted social habits of the day. Here psychoanalytic biographical interpretation (as with psychoanalytic clinical interpretation) depends on the art of listening—of listening as carefully as possible to the traces of the life, and of knowing the historical context as deeply as possible, so that one can hear the indi-vidual nuances one's subject is giving to the shared social and historical experiences of the times. It is also a matter of listening as carefully as possi-ble to one's own responses—both for clues as to the subject's emotions, and for warnings as to the possible interference of one's own psychological and emotional patterns. In biography psychoanalysis is more about practising an art than applying a scientific theory, and it can be done more or less well.

In tracing the inner life in the outer actions and events of a person's life, or the impact of outer experiences on the inner life, biographers are writing, in good part, about their subjects' emotions—their hates, loves and fears, their joys and griefs, their angers and triumphs, and so on. Psychoanalysis provides the biographer with a grammar of the emotions to guide this interpretative task. Psychoanalysis is the body of modern thought which has reflected in the most systematic and sustained way on human emotional life, producing theories about the relationships between various human emotions, and between experience and emotions. The term 'grammar of the emotions' conveys the way psychoanalysis is interested in emotional sequences and consequences, and in emotional exclusions and incompatibilities, for example in such relationships as those between envy and idealisation, anger and despair, fear of dependence and the propensity to blame. Psychoanalysis thus provides the biographer with theories which help guide their attempts to understand the conflicts and emotional dramas of their subject's life. Without it, the biographer has only the various understandings of the emotions embedded in common sense, in religious understandings and in literature. Common sense, religion and literature are all important sources for the understanding biographers bring to their subjects' emotional lives, but they are not systematic, and so do not provide a systematic guide with which to control one's reflection and intuitive hunches. Nor, I would argue, are they always as successful at penetrating the hidden logic of emotions, at revealing patterns not otherwise discernible.

In tracing the emotional patterns of a person's life the biographer is not necessarily revealing anything that is secret or hidden, but is rather simply tracing patterns across a life which are there for all to see if they can read the connections. This brings me to the very vexed questions of time and causation in psychoanalytically informed biography, and the relationship between the patterns of the adult life and the subject's childhood. One of the common points of resistance to psychoanalytic interpretations in biography is that it reduces the adult life to the playing out of childhood experience. Freud stressed the formative role of childhood in human life, not just as a stage through which we pass on our journey through life, but as a period which reverberates throughout life, as the child's relations within the family are transformed into the relationships and attachments of adult life. It is in the family that the child first confronts the constraints and the pleasures that make them a 'civilised' member of society. Children's relations with their parents are thus fundamentally and inevitably conflicted and ambivalent as the parents impose controls and meanings on their children's aggression, sexuality and narcissism.

The conflicts and ambivalences, the fears and anxieties, as well as the joys and intense pleasure of childhood retain their psychic reality into adult life. Many biographers seem to regard their subject's childhood as something for chapter one, with as much period detail as possible to disguise the often thin primary material. Such an approach leads, to my mind, to a thin adult life. The thicker and more real one can make the childhood, the richer will be the adult life. And to keep the childhood confined to chapter one obscures the continuing presence of childhood in the memory of the adult. The grown-up remembers they were once a child, even if some biographer may be tempted to forget. Graham Little stresses the need for the self of childhood and the self of adulthood to work out a story on which they can both agree.[12] Childhood has its uses for the adult—an excuse for later failures, a repository of wisdom or of innocence, a measure of the distance travelled ('look how far I've come . . .'), and so on.

Childhood also has its uses for biographers, who are generally writing about people older than themselves and who thus always run the risk of seeing them in the larger-than-life terms in which they once saw their own parents. To be reminded that one's subjects were once children helps to remind the biographer of the continuing vulnerabilities of the adult, and to provide a check on the temptation to turn their subjects into either villains or heroes.

These uses aside, however, the vexed question remains of the relationship between the experiences of childhood and adult life. Freud's work fundamentally altered our view of the relationship between childhood and adult life, but it did so within an essentially causal and determinist framework of thinking. As Juliet Mitchell puts it, Freud's 'historical imagination examines the present (the adult illness) and from it reconstructs a hypothetical past determinant'.[13] In Freud the past produces the present. It is just this point to which many people object; it can seem to reduce the achievements and the failures of the adult life to an epiphenomenon of some past event, often traumatic; it can seem to reduce the grown man or woman again to a little child; it can seem, almost, to wipe out adult life. Now these are oversimplifications of Freud, but nevertheless they are responding to the primacy which Freud gives to the past.

Many later psychoanalysts, however, in particular Melanie Klein and the British Object Relations School which developed from her work, operate with a quite different understanding of time—one in which past and present are one, in which psychological positions/constellations, first experienced in infancy, continue to exist as permanent possibilities in the adult psyche. From this perspective, psychoanalytic interpretations of adult life are not uncovering some past determinant of that life, but a present psychological reality in which past and present may share the same patterns, without the implication that the past caused the present. Juliet Mitchell again:

Klein is not a scientific theorist in the nineteenth-century tradition. The great theorists of the nineteenth century—Darwin, Marx and Freud—explain the present by the past. The dominant sociological phenomenologies of the twentieth century in which Klein participated study lateral, horizontal, not vertical relationships.[14]

Psychoanalytic interpretation can thus be understood as a matter not of digging up causes, but of revealing patterns—both within a particular slice of time and across time.

The English biographer Richard Holmes says of biography:

all biographers work essentially in a narrative mode—they tell the *story* of a life. Yet the truth they reveal is essentially figurative, the symbolic or representative elements within a life, and to that extent [a] timeless, transcending story . . . Partly this seems to me a question of biographers using two *kinds* of time. One is historical time, which produces chronology, 'the plot', the daily events of a life, set against their unfolding historical background. The other may be called interior time, the inner life of the subject, which makes patterns of impulse and imagery, repetitions and recollections, constellations of self-myth and self-understanding, links between childhood and adult experience, which obey the quite different, unhistorical, or 'dream laws' of memory and imagination.[15]

Add to this the Kleinian and the later object-relations theorists' attention to the traffic between inner and outer reality and you have what I see as the key contribution psychoanalysis can make to biography—attentiveness to the patterns of interaction between the inner and outer life. Although they are often right before one's nose, these patterns only reveal themselves when the biographer lifts their attention from the moving edge of time, the sequence of people and events which make up the subject's outer life, to an essentially spatial contemplation of the whole—the life spread out like a landscape, the biographer's eye roving back and forth for patterns and disruptions, evasions and telling absences, projects started but abandoned, self-defeating repetitions, recurrent strategies for success and obstacles surprisingly overcome.

There is one last point I want to make: some objections to the use of psychoanalysis by biographers are aesthetic rather than intellectual. Much psychoanalytic terminology is ugly; it introduces technical-sounding words into what is primarily a literary form and so disrupts certain of the pleasures of reading biography. Leon Edel, who is committed to the biographer using psychoanalysis to develop his understanding of his subject, counsels that, nevertheless, the biographer should eschew psychoanalytic terminology:

> Having arrived at an understanding of his subject he must now recreate him in words, and as a palpable, living being, in language proper to himself and to those who will read of him ... The main duty of the literary biographer, it seems to me, is to gain his insights, understand the motivations of his subject, and then cast aside this special language, bury completely the tools that have served him in attaining his ends. He must write as if psycho-analysis never existed.[16]

This is a perfectly defensible position, but it is motivated primarily by a romantic aesthetic. To embed one's interpretation in a good read seduces people into accepting as certainties what are, after all, only provisional, artful interpretations. Psychoanalytic interpretations are just that—interpretations. A biographer may well want to let the reader in on the making of them, to lay on the table the steps through which that interpretation was developed so that the reader can in part make up their own mind. This disrupts the identification of the reader with the subject of the biography, but that is the point. It must be admitted, however, that this is a risky strategy, for the more visible the psychoanalytic basis of the interpretation, the more the various preconceptions about psychoanalysis are aroused, preconceptions which can easily come between potential readers and the book.

Conclusion

Psychoanalysis begins from suspicion. It holds that things are not always as they seem, that people do not always say or even know what they mean, that human beings are not transparent to themselves or each other. In this core of suspicion psychoanalysis seems ideally suited to political biographers in the liberal tradition, in which one always has a weather-eye cocked for potential abuses of power. That it is not more popular is perhaps because it does not stay with suspicion and its comfortable bedfellow, cynicism, but moves on to compassion. For psychoanalysis also began in the quest to heal. Of course biographers are not in the business of healing, but those who use psychoanalysis are implicated in its quest to understand human lives in all their moral and emotional complexity. To look long and hard at a life, to remember that this person was once a vulnerable and dependent child, to realise that the person's achievements may only be possible because of their self-deceptions, to remember above all that this person is not a god or a saint or even a hero, but only a man or woman, is to refuse both denigration and idealisation. For those who want a world of villains and heroes psychoanalysis will never be convincing, but for those who want to understand political leaders and their quest for power it has much to offer.

7

Reading the Victorian family

John Rickard

I CANNOT REMEMBER what the first biography I ever read was. But I date my enthusiasm for the genre from an early encounter with Lytton Strachey's *Eminent Victorians*, which tantalised with the suggestion of the biographer's power to pry into the darker corners of his subjects' lives. Then there was Stefan Zweig: as a student I was particularly drawn to his study of that great survivor of the French Revolution, Joseph Fouché, who was fascinating simply because of 'his amazingly persistent lack of character—his unfailing want of principle'. Zweig concluded that 'it is just because he [Fouché] is an enigma that we of a later day are lured into an attempt to practice the art at which he himself excelled, the art of unravelling a mystery'.[1] What could be more seductive than the idea of the biographer as sleuth, particularly to a young reader who was a devotee of Hercule Poirot and Miss Marple? Zweig was also a friend and admirer of Freud,[2] though he did not in his biographies draw on psychoanalysis in any theorised sense. But Freud was in the air, if not the text. Many years later Michael Holroyd's seminal biography of Strachey brought me back full circle to my starting point, but with a new appreciation of the difference between a brilliant biographical sketch and a complex, full-scale portrait.

When, having left the role-playing of theatre behind me (I worked as an actor through the 1960s) I began teaching and writing history at Monash, I considered the possibility of turning biographer, the potential subject being H. B. Higgins, with whom I had become acquainted in the course of writing

Class and Politics.[3] A. F. (Foo) Davies had been good enough to read a draft of *Class and Politics* and from time to time I would drop in on the psychosocial seminar he presided over at the University of Melbourne. But, to tell the truth, although I was charmed by Davies (who some years later was to launch *H. B. Higgins: The Rebel as Judge*) I was rather intimidated by the self-conscious intellectual atmosphere of the seminar. But then, I was something of a psychoanalytical innocent.

About this time two notable historians, Frank Manuel and Saul Friedlander, gave papers at Monash which canvassed the use of psychoanalytical theory in biography and history.[4] I was excited by the possibilities they suggested, and in 1978, when I was planning to start writing up Higgins, I arranged to spend a few months at UCLA where Peter Loewenberg, a historian and analyst, was my host.[5] I sat in on some of his classes—the Austro-Marxists of the late nineteenth century were one of his preoccupations at the time—and, at his suggestion, I underwent what might be called a 'sample' analysis with a colleague of his.

So, precisely at the moment that I started to write the chapters dealing with Higgins's Irish childhood, I was going twice a week to Victor, beginning the journey into my own rather different childhood. The fact that this was occurring in the sometimes surreal atmosphere of Los Angeles, far from the Melbourne and Sydney of my early years, added to a feeling of dislocation. In telling my story to Victor there was at times a need for some kind of cultural translation.

In a city which offered a vast array of psychotherapies, Victor was pretty much a conventional Freudian. When we first met he offered me the choice of the couch or a chair. Resisting, I imagine, the notion that I was a patient, I opted for the chair, a decision which I later regretted but felt bound to stick with. Victor would fix me with his intense stare, and if my gaze wandered to the window he would comment on it. But mostly, of course, I just talked while Victor listened—I don't remember him taking notes—until as the end of the magic hour (or more precisely fifty minutes) was reached he would offer some interpretations or comments.

I usually came to my session armed with an agenda, very much as if I were preparing for a tutorial. I had entered a phase when I was remembering dreams much more than I am usually given to do and these I took some satisfaction in presenting to Victor. I was still wary of him—and there is a sense in which one cannot help but be wary of one's analyst—and almost felt some disloyalty to my parents in talking so intimately about them to this total (American) stranger. But one morning a particular dream I recounted seemed to trigger a chain reaction. He asked me what I made of the dream; I had an interpretation already prepared and he nodded in agreement—but then proceeded to identify a further layer of meaning which impressed me with its neatness. It rang true in a personal sense while simultaneously being intellectually satisfying.

I returned to Higgins that day feeling that I understood a little more about psychoanalysis, and turning to Higgins's unpublished memoir, read once more his account of his first memories of his Irish childhood. His first recollection is of his father, a Wesleyan preacher, on horseback, farewelling his three boys and riding off to an appointment, which is followed by two memories of childhood fear. The first involves Mr Humphreys, the local miller, 'a big, stout, masterful man', who made a playful threat to put the children in a dark coal room under the stairs, a threat which young Henry at least took seriously. He goes on:

> Another, but fascinating, terror was in the story which a lady visitor often repeated to me—the Spider and the Fly—'Will you walk into my parlour said the Spider to the Fly?' I always looked forward to what was coming: suiting the action to the word the lady would pounce on me to eat me, as the spider the fly. I became a 'delicate' child. I remember lying on my bed, and watching my mother and (I think) Bawdit preparing leeches to put on my face . . .[6]

It was with a tingle of excitement that I suddenly appreciated that what was at work here was free association. Although his first memory is of his father, it essentially records his absence. This is followed by two memories of fear and vulnerability, the first in the male form of the 'masterful' Humphreys, the second in the more insidious form of 'the lady visitor' who, although clearly well known in the Higgins household, is mysteriously unidentified. The story of the spider and the fly, with its cannibalistic climax, immediately leads him to recall that he became a 'delicate' child. The outward sign of his delicate health was a paralysing stammer which in later life he would struggle to overcome. But by placing the word 'delicate' in inverted commas Higgins throws up a question mark, implying that the condition was some-how imposed upon him. But if the infant Higgins is the fly in this regard, who is the real spider? The next memory shift provides the answer all too clearly: there is his mother, preparing leeches to put on his face. (Bawdit, the nickname for their maid who was almost a member of the family, is possibly present, but he is not sure.)

Once I had recognised the psychic connection between these apparently random thoughts, the interpretation seemed incontrovertible. And even now, all these years later, I can see small things which reinforce it. How, for example, the lady visitor pouncing on him, even while it was something he 'looked forward to', might easily provoke an excited, hysterical response which would have left him, so to speak, tongue-tied. And what of the parallel between the spider eating the fly and the leeches feeding on his face? As has been pointed out to me, there is also an erotic flavour to the memory.[7] The dependence of the 'delicate' child on the strong-willed, caring mother could be seductive, even while being a source of unconscious resentment.

A sceptic might see such an interpretation as reading too much into the evidence, but it is consistent with a more general mapping of family relationships based on a range of sources. In reading memoirs and autobiographies —particularly those written in a pre-Freudian era when subjects were not alert to the risks of psychological disclosure—it is sensible to keep an eye out for the function of free association. But it is also important to look for the repetitions in the text, because they can offer clues to the workings of the unconscious.

In Higgins's case, I was struck by a certain grim fascination he seemed to have with madness and mental disorders. There are several references in his memoir to encounters with people who were mentally inflicted: for example, a teacher at his school, initially recalled as a rather sinister figure, begins to pass into trance-like states and is taken away by his mother. But the theme is crystallised in one striking episode:

> One evening I happened to be alone in the house at Abbeyleix. I found an idiot boy, a familiar figure of the town, facing me. There used to be in Ireland a reverential feeling for persons so afflicted. They were treated as if they were wards of God himself. No one could injure them; no one would mock at them. Everyone would do them a kindness, if possible—the 'innocents' as they were called. The boy was harmless, and was easily removed.[8]

There is almost a surreal feeling to this incident. The idiot boy seems to materialise from nowhere, while at the end he is 'easily removed', though it is not clear by whom. And in spite of the cultural context given by Higgins concerning the respectful Irish attitude to 'persons so afflicted', there is a lurking sense of threat. Although the boy is 'harmless' he does need to be 'removed'.

Now elsewhere Higgins records how through the trials and tribulations of his ill health, he acquired a reputation for saintliness and gentleness in childhood, a reputation the adult Higgins was uneasy with. We must also bear in mind the effects of the humiliating stammer, of which he writes that 'no one who has not been afflicted with a stammer can realise the degradation which one feels who is afflicted'.[9] Having unravelled the story of the spider and the fly, I began to understand the significance of the nexus between saintliness and mental affliction, and to appreciate why the encounter with the idiot boy of Abbeyleix should have lodged itself so firmly in his memory. His reputation as a saintly child, reinforced by the 'affliction' of the stammer, finds an echo in the idiot boy: the encounter is unsettling simply because he is confronting a distorted image of himself. Higgins's unconscious concern was that those around him were treating him with the tenderness and reverence accorded the 'innocents'.

The adult Higgins was uneasy about his childhood saintliness simply because he knew it was unmerited, just as he sensed that his delicate health was not constitutional. By contrast, Higgins as a politician and public figure always sought to maintain an image of moral rectitude, as if to compensate for what in childhood he had not earned. The recurring theme of mental affliction in his memoir is therefore important, both for what it reveals about the traumas of his childhood as well as the development of his adult public persona. Repetitions may take many forms, but those with an emotional resonance (even if we cannot immediately identify its precise nature) warrant particular attention.

In the case of Higgins I was lucky as a biographer that there was not only his memoir written in old age but also family letters—some, for example, between his parents discussing their children—from the Irish period. So Higgins's recollections could sometimes be checked against contemporary accounts of significant events in the family's history. Similarly, one reason for being drawn to Alfred Deakin and his family was the very substantial collection of Deakin papers, supplemented by the much smaller, but very useful, collection left by his sister Catherine.[10]

J. A. La Nauze published the important, standard biography of Deakin in 1965. Back then it was regarded as a historical landmark, helping to establish the academic respectability of biography at a time when many historians did not see the particularity of biography—the life of one person—as consistent with the generalisations required of 'real' history. *Alfred Deakin* was essentially a political biography, but, given the riches of the sources, La Nauze could hardly afford to ignore Deakin's well-documented inner life or his family relationships. Uncomfortable with Deakin's interest in spirituality—and spiritualism—La Nauze's solution was to safely quarantine this material in chapter three ('"Insights", Prayer and Praise') with the hope, it would seem, that it would not contaminate the main narrative. As for family relationships, La Nauze's brief sketch threw out one tantalising morsel which was to be the starting point for my own book:

> As a young man he [Deakin] was consulted, by one known to himself and his sister, about her likely attitude to a proposal of marriage. Without in turn consulting her, he took it on himself firmly to discourage it. The would-be suitor in time married another; only later did Deakin learn that his beloved sister would happily have welcomed the proposal.[11]

La Nauze, usually such a stickler for documentation, gave no source for this story, which I assumed came from family oral tradition. It seemed remarkable that Alfred could have taken it upon himself to deflect the unknown suitor, and it raised all sorts of questions about the relationship between Catherine, who was to remain a spinster, and her precocious younger brother. Brother and sister were very close: indeed, Catherine began a reminiscence written after Alfred's death with the unequivocal declaration that 'I worshipped the baby as I have the man during all our lives'.[12] As I delved into the papers of Alfred and Catherine I came to appreciate the complex triangle of relationships that developed when Alfred married the young and beautiful Pattie Browne. All this was in the extraordinary context of the spiritualist movement in which they were involved: indeed Alfred, at the age of twenty-two, was president of the Victorian Association of Progressive Spiritualists, while Pattie had already won renown as a child medium.

I was concerned from the beginning that the spiritualist phenomena which were so important for Alfred, Pattie and Catherine had to be, in a biographical sense, taken seriously. But psychoanalysis offered some interesting perspectives on the psychic significance of their spiritualist experiences. The outstanding example is provided by Alfred's remarkable text, privately published, which was the product of séances conducted over something like a year. Alfred had already shown some capacity as a medium, and in the weekly séance presided over by one of Melbourne's most respected spiritualists, Dr Motherwell, the pencil in Alfred's hand dashed across the page, in the practice known as passive or automatic writing, giving forth the spiritualist allegory, *A New Pilgrim's Progress*, which Alfred at the time believed was dictated by the spirit of John Bunyan.[13] Deakin was not identified as the author: the text was described on the title page as 'purporting to be given through an impressional writing medium'. *A New Pilgrim's Progress* was very different from Bunyan's allegory, but there was a real sense in which it was inspired by it: for it hardly comes as a surprise that *A Pilgrim's Progress* had been one of young Alfred's favourite books.

La Nauze could not ignore this extraordinary document, but he was clearly embarrassed by it, treating it as a piece of juvenilia. He conceded that the depiction of the central character, Restless (who later becomes Redeemer), could reflect 'the wishful thinking of Deakin the undergraduate'. And he goes on:

> There is much more in this curious book that may—or may not—explain something about its author other than that he was a gifted youth, in some danger of assuming that he had a mission. There may be reflections of his feelings for Pattie Browne, then about fourteen, in the gentle maiden Wilful (later Redemptress) whom Restless protects, and later marries.[14]

What La Nauze is hinting at here, the biographer drawing on Freud can state boldly: if, as Deakin himself did in later years, we discount the possibility of Bunyan having had a hand in *A New Pilgrim's Progress*, we have here a document which is the creation of young Alfred's unconscious. In the spiritual journey of Restless we can see the process of identity formation being played out.

What is particularly remarkable about *A New Pilgrim's Progress* is the way it prefigures Alfred's relationship with Pattie. Like Pattie, Wilful is a powerful medium, and there is much in her character that is suggestive of Pattie. At the time of its writing, Alfred would have been aware of the child medium who was considered something of a prodigy in spiritualist circles. She was also a pupil at the Progressive Lyceum, the spiritualist Sunday school where Alfred was a teacher. A year or two after its publication the principal medium in Dr Motherwell's séance circle, Mrs Loudon, confirmed that Pattie, who would have then been about fifteen or sixteen, was his 'predestined mate'.[15] When Pattie turned eighteen Alfred began to court her and they were married, against her parents' wishes, a year later. But the blueprint for their relationship had already been laid out in *A New Pilgrim's Progress*. Although in later years both Alfred and Pattie moved away from an active interest in spiritualism, and although Alfred, at least, came to doubt the spiritualist authenticity of the document which his hand had produced, *A New Pilgrim's Progress* retained a special place in the story of their romance and marriage. It is striking that while La Nauze could hint at this, he did not feel able as a biographer to pursue the inquiry. The unconscious was out of bounds for the historian.

The Higgins and Deakin families were different in many respects. The former originally comprised eight children, all of whom were born in Ireland; in the latter, by contrast, there were just Catherine and Alfred, both born in Australia of immigrant parents. But it is notable that in both families sibling relationships played a crucial role. Henry and Alfred were the second born in their families, and both were cast in significant relationships with their elder siblings. In Henry's case it was a competitive and ultimately tragic relationship; with Alfred and Catherine it was more complex, yet also had unhappy consequences.

Henry's brother James was two years his elder and was considered something of a ne'er-do-well. Higgins himself describes his brother as being 'impetuous, lively, repugnant to regular discipline; and often in trouble'.[16] To us his sins might seem relatively minor, but he fell short of the moral values demanded of him by his parents and by the Wesleyan Connexional School in Dublin to which, as a minister's son, he was sent. When Henry followed his brother to the school, the contrast between them was firmly established: the 'incorrigible' James, who seemed constitutionally unable to bring home a certificate of good conduct, could now be compared with the well-behaved, conscientious Henry. James was not without charm or, as he grew into a youth, good looks; but, conscious of his own shortcomings, he was prone to remorse and self-doubt. Henry was shy, awkward and still sickly, but firmly committed to living up to the good reputation he enjoyed.

What the headmaster described as an 'unpleasantness' between James and one of the masters led to his being withdrawn from the school. What to do with James became a worrying concern for his parents. The ultimate solution seems to have been chosen by James himself: the classic Irish way out—emigration. At the age of seventeen he set off on his own for New York. Emigration had long been a subject for discussion, and it is possible that James was being given the opportunity to be the advance guard for the family. From New York he wrote vivid, enthusiastic letters home conveying the excitement of the New World. Although his letters were, as Henry put it, 'brimming over with affection' (that phrase suggesting a reservation concerning James's sincerity), he seemed to relish the freedom of the new life.[17] But the escape from Ireland was short-lived. He fell ill with consumption and returned to Ireland virtually an invalid. His death in 1869 prompted the decision to migrate, but the United States was now off the agenda. Victoria was recommended for its healthy climate.

I was much struck by the relationship between the two brothers—given here in capsule form—and before finishing the book felt moved to write an article on 'poor James', as he came to be called, trying to imagine his side of the story.[18] He was one of history's discards, yet his letters from New York were fascinating and revealing documents, suggesting both the strength of family ties and James's need to escape them. But I also came to appreciate the importance of James's death in Higgins's life. For while Henry had been the delicate child and sometimes pampered accordingly, it was the wayward James who was the ultimate victim. There was a sense in which Henry's reputation for virtue had contributed to his brother's fall from grace. James's death meant that Henry was now the eldest son, and on the journey to Australia he had a foretaste of being the head of the family, as his father remained in Ireland for a further six months to complete his term on the Wesleyan circuit. There was a final irony which Higgins himself could not bring himself to point out in his memoir: James died on 30 June 1869, which happened to be young Henry's eighteenth birthday.

But, in a sense, James lived on, even in distant Australia. The death of James and the kind of guilt that Higgins might have felt over it help explain his adult uneasiness with his childhood reputation for saintliness. The extent to which James featured in his memoir, written more than fifty years later, provides ample evidence of the importance of Henry's dead brother. Once again, a careful psychological reading of this document was called for. It was even relevant to note the passages where Higgins had made more corrections than usual, as if having difficulty finding the right words for his emotions.

But there were other indicators. At a time of great trauma during World War I, following the death of his only son Mervyn and when the death of Henry's indomitable mother was being expected, he circulated James's letters from New York to younger members of the family. It was as if the guilt a father might feel for the death of a son reminded him of that earlier death, and this was reinforced by the suggestion that there were aspects of Mervyn which reminded him of James.

Was it fanciful, too, to point to the way in which Higgins seemed drawn to the theme of rivalry between brothers? For example he was fascinated by the Promethean myth, and as a literary exercise made his own translation of the Aeschylus text, *Prometheus Bound*. In the beginning the relationship between Zeus and Prometheus is fraternal in character; but when Prometheus steals fire from Olympus and presents it as a gift to the human race, he is punished by Zeus and chained to a rock where an eagle feeds daily on his liver. Ultimately, however, Zeus and Prometheus are reconciled. Then in one of his judgments in the Arbitration Court, Higgins identified the weakness of labour's bargaining position in these terms: 'The worker is in the same position, in principle, as Esau, when he surrendered his birthright for a square meal'.[19] Again Higgins was invoking a conflict between brothers. Esau and Jacob are twins, but Esau is the first born. In the biblical story Jacob is the usurper, stealing his brother's birthright and their father's blessing. But Jacob redeems himself and the brothers are finally reunited. In the biography I drew attention to the Promethean character of Higgins's mission in industrial arbitration, but I wanted also to suggest that in identifying with Prometheus and, by implication, with Jacob, he was coming to terms with a sense of guilt stemming from his unhappy relationship with James.

In the case of Alfred Deakin the relationship with his sister Catherine was to have repercussions beyond their own generation. As a girl Catherine had been devoted to her baby brother and was much involved in caring for him, but as he matured into a handsome, personable youth the nature of their relationship changed. 'We went out a great deal together', Catherine recalled, 'and received a great many visitors in a quiet way for croquet and dancing.'[20] Although she retained a degree of authority attached to the role of elder sister she now increasingly deferred to her brilliant brother, particularly as his precocious public career unfolded, first in the spiritualist movement, and then in politics.

The relationship necessarily changed again when Alfred married Pattie. Although the Brownes were well-off, the disapproval of the match on the part of her parents meant that she brought no dowry with her. For a year or so the young couple lived with the Deakin family, and it seemed marvellously symbolic that Catherine gave up her bedroom to them in the modest South Yarra home. In his fifties Alfred confessed in a journal to feeling 'inappeasable shame and regret' for one unspecified incident in his life and it is likely that he was referring to his thoughtless presumption in deflecting Catherine's suitor.[21] We do not know if Catherine was aware of her young brother's extraordinary intervention in her life. I suspect that she was not, which would only have added to Alfred's burden of guilt. It meant that he felt a particular responsibility towards her, and he maintained a close relationship with his sister for the rest of his life, always stressing his continuing debt to her. He committed the education of his three daughters to her, and this in turn eventually led to a falling out between Catherine and Pattie, who came to resent Catherine's role in the bringing up of her children. Although initially papered over, the schism grew wider with time, and after Alfred's death they were totally alienated from each other. It also affected the relationship between the three daughters, Ivy, Stella and Vera, whose loyalties were divided. Recently, revisiting the Deakin family story when writing an article on Vera Deakin White for the *Australian Dictionary of Biography*, I found myself reflecting on the way in which family dramas decades later could be traced back to their source in that simple, destructively foolish act of Alfred's. Why did he do it? In *A Family Romance* I offered some speculations. As a young woman Catherine had enjoyed poor health and child bearing might have been thought inadvisable. It is also possible that as the only daughter there was an expectation that she would remain in the household to take care of their parents. I also suggest a more complex scenario.[22]

Catherine was an accomplished pianist and musician; she was also well-read, sharing with Alfred many of his intellectual and cultural interests. Throughout his political career he treated her as a confidant, and when the split with Pattie made it difficult for Catherine to be received in their home he called on her regularly. For Catherine, the relationship with her successful brother offered her a window onto the world. Even after his marriage Catherine met interesting and important people through her brother, and she was able to feel that she could give Alfred the intellectual support which Pattie was less capable of. The disappointments of her own life and the extent to which her career as a teacher had been contained within the family were compensated for by the vicarious access which Alfred's career gave her to the public sphere.

There is more than an echo of this in Higgins's relationship with his younger sister, Ina, who, like Catherine, was a spinster. Ina had her own life and interests—she was something of a feminist, and studied horticulture at Burnley College—but she also invested much in her brother's career. She was immensely proud of Henry, and followed his career closely. Higgins recognised her loyalty and understanding of his achievements when he left his papers to her. In this brother and sister relationship there were none of the tensions which were attached to Catherine's devotion to Alfred. Ina was much loved and respected in the wider Higgins family. But there was one family drama which caused her pain. Ina was very fond of their nephew Esmonde, the younger brother of Nettie Palmer. In the wake of World War I Esmonde, a disillusioned idealist, embraced communism, and wrote a very critical review of his uncle's apologia for his life's work in arbitration, *A New Province for Law and Order*.[23] Ina, herself something of a socialist, reprimanded Esmonde for his 'senseless, ill natured attack'—but she did not, as it were, disown him.[24] Esmonde's communism also caused problems for his relationship with his sister, Nettie, and we can see here, in the next generation, another version of the intense sister–brother relationship being played out.

Although the relationship between Henry and James Higgins was contained within a large family, in which a variety of sibling alliances was possible, the implicit rivalry between the two brothers was highlighted by their isolation from the rest of the family at the Wesleyan Connexional School. James's sad death was the final trigger for emigration: later the family could look back and see 'poor James' as being part of the unhappy Ireland they had left behind. But, as I have suggested, for Henry, James lived on—as, indeed, did Ireland, and with the death of his only son in World War I Higgins's thoughts turned more and more to the land of his birth, culminating in the remarkable legacy to the Royal Irish Academy which dominated his will. It was as if he was repaying his debt to 'poor James'.

For Catherine and Alfred, on the other hand, the fact that they were the only two children intensified their relationship. It was a close-knit, loving family, but there was a sense in which daughter and son, with the benefit of a good education, left their immigrant parents behind. As much as they were devoted to their parents—particularly their loyal and caring mother—their sibling relationship also served to exclude them. I am still surprised by the unembarrassed passion of Catherine's declaration: 'I worshipped the baby as I have the man during all our lives'. One has to appreciate how the Victorian family could accommodate such powerful emotion. It is true enough that, given the limitations placed on women in terms of education and career, the relationship of sister to brother could take on special importance. And while for the sister the relationship offered access to the public sphere, for the brother there was the emotional benefit of an intimate relationship with a woman that was not inhibited by the rituals of courtship. Yet Catherine's considered choice of the word 'worship'—the reminiscence was written for Walter Murdoch, Deakin's first biographer—still strikes me as remarkable.[25]

It is a truism to say that Freudian psychoanalysis was a product of late nineteenth-century Viennese culture and that its precepts need to be understood in that context. But it is important to recognise that the dynamics of the Victorian family were often different from those we are used to today. And in an immigrant community the comparative lack of extended families —a shortage of aunts and uncles and cousins as it were—needs to be noted. We are accustomed to regarding the Victorian family as a rather oppressive institution, hidebound and morally censorious. At first sight neither the Higgins nor Deakin families fits this model. But both families inhabited a middle-class culture with clear understandings of what constituted accept-able and appropriate behaviour—and of what could be said and not said. The restrictions placed on behaviour meant that language often carried a greater responsibility as a bearer of emotion. And within the bounds of the topics which could be addressed (particularly by women) emotion could be given full reign; indeed the culture often encouraged the fervent expression of such emotion. Peter Gay speculates that 'the century of Victoria was at heart more profoundly erotic than ages more casual about their carnal desires and consummations'.[26] In entering the world recorded in the journals and letters of the Victorians we need to recognise the different emotional land-scape, and in interpreting these documents take care to respect the signifi-cance of the messages they convey.

8

'I knew I would be lonely for them always': Donald Thomson and campaigns for Aboriginal rights

Bain Attwood

IN EARLY JANUARY 1947 Australian anthropologist Donald Thomson received a letter from Bill Onus, President of the Australian Aborigines' League, seeking his help. Usually a poor correspondent, Thomson hastened to respond to his fellow Melburnian; after thanking the Aboriginal leader for his 'generous remarks' about Thomson's recent newspaper articles on Aboriginal rights, he quickly went on:

> I would be very happy to feel that these have given to your League new impetus in its fight. I write now to assure you of my goodwill and backing in your efforts to get justice and liberty for your people for whom I have a great regard and admiration. Perhaps I can make you understand my feelings most easily by saying that I wish that I myself were an Aborigine so that I had the right to fight with you . . .
>
> May I suggest that, in making your plea for liberty and freedom . . . you make your first objective and ideal the development of a racial pride among your people, that you teach them to be proud of their own background and culture . . .
>
> I know the people of Cape York Peninsula and Arnhem Land well. I have lived with them for years and learned to love and to respect them. They applied their own kinship or relationship terms to me, because I am proud to say they regarded me as one of themselves, not as a 'white man' but just as fellow human being.
>
> You have a fine heritage, none the less great because few white men appear to be capable of understanding it. Your people are generous and tolerant and they know what altruism is.[1]

Donald Thomson often expressed both his love for 'aborigines' and his desire to be an Aboriginal person. On leaving north-east Arnhem Land ten years earlier he confided in his diary: 'I . . . realised . . . I knew and loved the Arnhem Land people and that I had more in common with them than with my own kind. I knew I would be lonely for them always.'[2]

In recent years Thomson has attracted the attention of scholars, particularly anthropologists looking to redeem their discipline in the context of postcolonial challenges. He has been represented as a progressive figure for his times, at the forefront of championing indigenous rights and passionately committed to Aboriginal people. Indeed in the middle decades of the twentieth century when Aboriginal policy came to be dominated by the goals of assimilation and equal rights, his championing of the ideals of Aboriginality and Aboriginal rights was a rare thing. Similarly, his representation of Aboriginal people has been commended: he presented them 'as individuals and active agents' which 'few other [contemporary] writings [did]' and recorded 'their interpretations' of the colonial world and 'their own reaction to their historical predicament'. This has been attributed to the fact he spent long periods in the field and to his relationships with Aboriginal people being 'close' and 'personal', informed by a 'desire to understand their society' and 'respect' for them.[3]

Thus far, however, scholars have not considered the origins of Thomson's exceptional advocacy nor indeed those of any other non-indigenous advocate or campaigner for Aboriginal rights, even though 'the Aboriginal cause' has undoubtedly attracted 'outsiders, eccentrics, [and] obsessive personalities'.[4] There seems to be a reluctance to do so, perhaps because historians are fearful of discovering 'just how deeply private emotions are invested in public life'.[5] Yet this is to foreclose upon a deeper understanding of many advocates and campaigns for indigenous rights as well as the nature of racial structures and representations. Towards this end, I consider here the ways in which Thomson's idealisation of, identification with, and advocacy for Aboriginal people reflected his own emotional investments.

Donald Thomson was first attracted to anthropological study of Aboriginal culture in his mid-twenties, and his turn to anthropology can best be understood in terms of his earlier interests. As a young boy he was attracted to natural history and developed a passion for collecting plants, observing animals and birds and recording their characteristics. In a youthful essay he wrote of 'the call of nature', describing it as a source for purification, strength and inspiration 'amid the drudgery of everyday life'; 'the bush' represented, it seems, a pleasurable escape from realities in the human world Thomson found unbearable. Later, at the University of Melbourne, he studied natural science—zoology and botany—and dreamed of joining a scientific expedition to a remote frontier. Upon completing his degree in 1925 he turned down an academic position for a cadetship in journalism that he hoped would pave the way to do expeditionary work. This opportunity came a few years later. In 1926 he sought Australian National Research Council (ANRC) funding to do anthropological research. A. R. Radcliffe Brown, Professor of Anthropology at the University of Sydney, told him he needed to get some training and enabled him to do a one-year course in his department in 1927. In the following year Thomson undertook several months of research on the remote north Australian frontier of Cape York and returned there shortly afterwards for a further and longer stint of fieldwork.[6]

Thomson reported this research in two long series of feature articles for newspapers. On the face of it there is little indication in these of the role he would later assume as an impassioned champion of Aboriginal rights: his account of settlers' cruel dispossession and treatment of Indigenous people, his consideration of the role of anthropological study, and his claim of colonial responsibility to and for Aboriginal people articulated sentiments commonly expressed by humanitarians and anthropologists at this time. Similarly, there was much that was conventional in the way he represented Aboriginal peoples and culture, as he echoed the evolutionary doctrines promulgated by imperial and colonial anthropology since the 1870s. Yet there are some clues in these articles and they are to be found through a closer reading of his representations of Aboriginal culture and a consideration of his accounts of his place on the frontiers of white settlement.

Anthropology was, of course, informed by the conviction that indigenous peoples were fundamentally 'other', but in Thomson's case this was unusually pronounced. He represented 'aborigines' as noble savages, a primitive people living in a benevolent state of nature. 'There is', he wrote several years later, 'some indefinable, permanent quality about these nomad hunters that abides in the memory. I, for one, cannot bear to think of their passing, these lithe, gentle, splendid, unspoiled primitive men, from their last little stronghold in the oldest Continent'. Thomson, I would argue, projected onto Aboriginal people and culture a fantasy of the world he wanted—an idyll where man was free and man and nature were at one. Aborigines, in his words, were 'happy nomads' for whom 'freedom [was] life', and 'the relationship of man with Nature [was] tempered with a mystic quality, and merge[d] into a dream world of magic and spirits'.[7]

Thomson felt he had found the place he so much wanted on the frontier and among Aboriginal people. On the one hand he enjoyed the romantic, idealised and masterful role he wrote for himself as the heroic explorer, on the other the place in the kinship systems he had been given, and the 'bond' and the 'staunch friends[hip]' this provided him. Most importantly, he had gained 'the confidence of the old men' and his chief informant addressed him as 'son' and he in turn called him 'father'. Significantly, he ascribed to Aborigines the qualities of tolerance and altruism and revealed that his 'own experience of the faithfulness of the blackfellow has been a particularly vivid and happy one'. He apparently relished the absence of conflict with his fellows, enjoying (in Inga Clendinnen's words) 'the security of uncontested because uncontestable inequality' the colonial racial hier-archy provided him.[8] This gave him the sense of union he was seeking. As such, Cape York was a haven or sanctuary for him—and so, not surpris-ingly, he called it 'home'. Indeed he became so absorbed by this world he 'los[t] touch with outside things altogether' and on returning to 'civilisation' had 'a sense of unreality, as if [he] had dropped too suddenly into a strange and unfamiliar world'.[9]

There were other ways, though, in which Thomson identified with Aboriginal people. To understand this, we must turn to events that occurred in December 1932 during his third field trip to Cape York, which proved a transforming experience in his life. At Aurukun, a Presbyterian mission station where Thomson and his wife, Gladys, spent eight months in 1932–33, he witnessed the arrest of several Aboriginal people by police at the direction of the autocratic superintendent, Bill MacKenzie. According to Thomson's account, three men and two women were 'chained and hand-cuffed in the Mission yard' before being 'driven' by two 'police troopers'—the men 'chained with heavy chains, neck to neck', the women 'following the police on horseback'. They travelled 'hundreds of miles' in 'tropical midsummer' heat to a township near Cooktown, where they were 'sent away' to Palm Island, a 'Penal Settlement' for Aborigines, thus being 'con-demned without trial, on the mere word of MacKenzie, to lifelong exile and imprisonment'. Thomson also observed men and women being 'thrown . . . into . . . iron cells' that had been 'devised . . . for the breaking of men' where they were 'chained to the corner posts'; young women being 'tied to trees . . . stripped and flogged with horsewhips'; and children being confined to 'a galvanised iron shed . . . like a gaol'. On his return to Melbourne, Thomson, a church-going Presbyterian, went to a 'counsellor and friend', a senior figure in the Church, D. K. Picken, the Master of Ormond College at the Uni-versity of Melbourne, and presented this account. But Picken proved un-sympathetic and he was refused a hearing by the Church.[10]

There can be no doubting either the importance of these events or Thomson's investment in them. Most immediately, he recorded the details in images and words, taking several photographs and then writing lengthy and detailed explanations of them, and on his return to Melbourne began to write about Aboriginal people much more personally and forcefully than ever before. For example he called the history of 'Australia's contact with, and administration of, the Aborigines one of failure', claiming it had 'not only resulted in the extinction of the majority of those with whom we have come into contact, but also of the *degradation* of the survivors [emphasis added]'. More to the point, in a newspaper article dealing with his time on Cape York, he claimed:

> I have never ceased to resent the treatment that we have meted out—and are still meting out not least in Queensland—to the Blackfellow. If I am able to help materially to bring about a better understanding between the aborigine and the white man, I feel I shall not have lived in vain. He is entitled to a better fate than to have his culture *systematically broken down*, and to end his days as a *despised hanger-on* of the white man [emphasis added].[11]

In subsequent years, Thomson returned again and again to this terrifying fantasy, describing Aurukun as 'a veritable hell'. He wrote most openly and at greatest length to Charles Duguid, a senior figure in the very church that had refused him a hearing and an older man willing to be a more accepting 'father'. In 1946 in the first of these letters, which he himself recognised or admitted was 'in the nature of a confession', Thomson wrote:

> I went into the field a young man with a keen sense of justice and fair play. And you know what I saw on a certain mission station, natives ill-used as I have never seen them ill-used and persecuted elsewhere . . . I saw these deportations of natives in chains by mounted police—driven by mounted police, without trial . . . I saw armed police driving natives on foot—manacled to exile on Palm Island.

Thomson also repeatedly described or invoked these events in features and opinions for the press, even when it was scarcely relevant or appropriate; in 1950, for example, he wrote an article in which he described events at Aurukun as a 'sight terrible to behold—and a memory that time will not expunge'.[12]

The material reality of the terrible oppression at Aurukun notwithstanding, there can little doubt this event was critical for Thomson because it had immense psychic significance for him.[13] To understand this we must first remind ourselves of the meaning of a place like Cape York for Thomson. This was, in his mind, paradise. In 1934 he sought to recapture this by describing his return to this imagined place: 'a great peace descended upon me. I was coming home. It is good to look upon a happy place, to be among friends, and to look upon a friendly place. As soon as the cutter crossed the bar of the river, a great shout went up, "Thomson come!"'. But in December 1932 the very antithesis to this world intruded in the form of MacKenzie and the police, plunging Thomson into a state of panic and despair.[14]

This was so because it provoked memories of an earlier trauma—fearful childhood conflicts, especially with his father, in which Thomson felt frustrated and humiliated. At Aurukun the slightly built Thomson once more felt himself impotent in the face of other, more powerful men, especially MacKenzie.[15] The missionary, he bitterly complained, acted in a cruel, arbitrary and authoritarian manner. Moreover, this patriarchal figure had such 'absolute control' that there were no means of redress or relief; the Aboriginal prisoners, he concluded, 'not only had no friend and protector, but were betrayed by their own Minister'.[16]

The neck chaining of the men, however, was the principal event in Thomson's mind, perhaps because it awakened memories of his own experience as a child when he was probably required to wear a neckbrace as treatment for curvature of the spine. He primarily identified with the men rather than with the women who were arrested, and over many years his accounts of the incident emphasised how the Aboriginal men had been 'manacled'. The removal and restraining of the children in dormitories—and there can be no doubting his identification with Aboriginal children separated from their parents—re-enacted, moreover, Thomson's childhood confinement to bed for diphtheria and a stint at boarding school. The removal of the adults symbolised his worse childhood fears of abandonment or exile: he reported an Aboriginal man named Donald had been removed the previous year and died 'on the road from cruelty and privations'.[17]

As a consequence of this situation Thomson, it seems reasonable to speculate, felt 'despised' and 'broken down', and this resulted in an emotionally powerful identification with a new object—not now just the realm of nature, but Aborigines, the most dispossessed of peoples. Their plight became his or, more accurately, his became theirs. This is evident in the way Thomson came to represent the historical situation of Aborigines. He attributed to them his own mental condition and projected his anxieties and needs onto them. Repeatedly he described Aboriginal culture as a fragile world that had been or would be destroyed by contact with an unfriendly outside (white) world with which it was incompatible. This object could only be protected by a radical measure—segregation in inviolable reserves where nobody except anthropologists and a few others could enter. The notion of Aborigines as a dying race was undoubtedly a common trope and segregation a common solution, but Thomson invested much more in this solution than other writers and continued to advocate this after most humanitarians became pro-assimilation in the late 1930s.[18]

Thomson tried to rid himself of the disturbing tensions produced by Aurukun by assuming the position of the Aborigines' champion. As we have seen, he first prepared a record of what had happened there in the hope it would be a powerful weapon in the fight for justice, but not long after he begged the Chancellor of the University of Melbourne to offer his services to the Commonwealth government as an 'intermediary' and adviser in the Northern Territory where, in a situation that paralleled the removal of the Aboriginal people at Cape York, Aboriginal men had been arrested and incarcerated for the killing of Japanese fishermen and a white police-man.[19] Powerful supporters at the university emphasised his passionate commitment and experience in pressing his case as an anthropological adviser and eventually they persuaded the government to appoint him as a patrol officer.[20]

Thomson was overjoyed by this restoration to the place he craved. He proposed to government that he could act as 'a special magistrate or arbi-trator in all matters concerning natives', triumphantly claiming magical, omnipotent powers: he 'would be to the natives a Protector in the full sense of the word.' Central to this rescue fantasy was a request Thomson imme-diately made when offered the position: that the *three* men imprisoned in Darwin for the killing of the Japanese fishermen be released to him so he could return them home. Contemplating his task more generally, Thomson believed he was 'going to know these people as few others have known them', claiming this would enable him 'to place their case before the Govern-ment more tellingly that any other advocate ha[d] been able to do'. In this regard he not only presented his role in the terms anthropologists had been asserting some time: that is, that their knowledge could assist government with 'native administration'. Thomson also claimed he had special expertise since he not only had the theoretical knowledge but also understood and knew Aborigines better than anyone else and so could 'obtain . . . the black man's point of view' and represent this both to governments and people, thus bringing about what Thomson believed the Aborigines (like himself) most needed: sympathy and understanding.[21]

Between 1935 and 1937 Thomson spent two long periods in north-east Arnhem Land, for the most part undertaking anthropological fieldwork, but regarding himself as a special commissioner for the Federal govern-ment. He again immersed himself in understanding an Aboriginal world and attached himself to its bearers. This understanding rested to a large degree upon his identification with the people of this area, the Yolngu, and on trying to see colonisation through their eyes. As a result of this, he believed they came to accept that he would be their mouthpiece 'in explain-ing their disadvantages and wrongs'. As he returned to 'civilisation' in 1937, however, Thomson was panicked by the realisation that he now had to convince the government and settler Australians of the need for a new Aboriginal policy. As it transpired, his recommendations—which principally consisted of a call for segregation of Indigenous Australians on inviolable reserves—were rejected by the Commonwealth government. These were far too radical since they envisaged the continuation of independent and separate Aboriginal communities in white Australia and entailed the valorisation of another culture. With the dismissal of his proposals, Thomson felt he had been spurned. 'There is nothing more than I can do here', he complained, 'I am going to England, and I do not think I will come back.'[22]

Shortly afterwards Thomson took up a Rockefeller Fellowship at the University of Cambridge but clearly still had high though misplaced hopes he might be appointed to a newly created post of Federal Commissioner for Native Affairs. During World War II he set these ambitions aside, but as his distinguished military service came to an end in 1943–44 his desire to champion the cause of Aboriginal people and assume control of Aboriginal affairs again became apparent. The rejection of his policy recommendations and his pleas for office in 1937–39 gnawed at him and fuelled his work over the following few years. In a series of writings he articulated the same ideals he had presented since his conversion to the Aboriginal cause. He continued to cast his role as that of an anthropologist whose task was one of confronting racial prejudice and increasing understanding. Because of his identification with Aboriginal people, he had considerable insight not only into Aboriginal cultures but also the nature of racism and its consequences. By increasing understanding Thomson hoped there would be pressure on governments for change, and he called repeatedly for 'a complete change of attitude on the part of the Commonwealth Government' and 'a complete overhaul of native policy'. In these years (and beyond) Thomson increasingly reasoned and argued in these stark, absolutist terms, repeating these polemical calls again and again.

More often than not, his prescriptions were very general. 'What is required', he asserted, was the right of Aborigines 'to work out [their] own destiny' and to live as 'free human beings', independent of white 'vested interests' and compulsion of any kind, 'political, economic and religious'. This demand for what Thomson called 'freedom and fair play' constituted, in his favourite phrase, 'justice for Aborigines'. It was, it can be argued, a personal dream rendered as a political ideal, and is best explained in terms of Thomson's own mental world. Certainly there is little indication in his innumerable writings that he drew on a body of abstract political principles or doctrines.[23]

This said, Thomson did develop something like a political program between 1944 and 1947, the result of his building upon North American indigenous policy (with which he had become acquainted while visiting there in 1939), proposals stimulated by the Atlantic Charter, and policies drawn up by left-wing activists Tom Wright and Brian Fitzpatrick. In a six-point plan in 1946 and a refined ten-point agenda the following year, Thomson rejected the policy of assimilation for those he called 'aborigines' —meaning 'tribal' Aborigines—which he saw as 'breaking up [indigenous] cultural, social and economic organisation'. He recommended 'an entirely new policy' that would recognise their rights 'to retain their own languages, ceremonies, traditions and culture' and provide for collective land owner-ship, indigenous courts, and a role in governing themselves.[24]

By contrast, Thomson's program for those who were generally called 'half-castes' echoed that of practically every white reformer of the day. He contended these peoples should be helped 'to adapt themselves to life as Australian citizens' and 'take a place . . . in white society.' He denied they were Aboriginal people; 'with the people of mixed blood there can only be one policy', he wrote in 1945, that of 'ultimate absorption', for they 'are not aborigines and cannot be treated as such. They must be treated as white men'. Only those 'still in possession of their own culture and way of life' had a legitimate claim to be Aboriginal and an entitlement to Aboriginal rights. Thomson's blinkered approach sprang from the fact that he had no experience of Aboriginal people in settled Australia, and so was ignorant of both cultural continuity and their sense of themselves as 'Aboriginal'; in other words, the kind of contact and imaginary space that led to his identi-fication with Aborigines in northern Australia and his articulation of in-digenous rights for *them* was absent.[25]

During 1946 and 1947 Thomson had forums to push his program, but he was becoming less and less a political player and increasingly withdrew from public life. His political role in the 1930s had depended upon his personal relationships with powerful father figures who acted as agents for him. Without their help he was politically incapacitated, the result of a con-viction that he lacked the personal resources required to fight for and defend his policies, as well as himself, in the rough and tumble of the world. His experience of political defeat in the 1930s aggravated this, leaving him with a (guilty) sense of having been 'able to achieve very little' and 'look-ing on ineffectively at a very terrible tragedy that [was] being enacted', and a (paranoid) sense he had made 'many enemies and . . . been branded as a crank and rebel'. In response to requests for help (like that of Onus), he would repeatedly pledge his commitment to the Aboriginal cause and promise his assistance but refuse public engagements and any involvement in political actions.[26]

Furthermore, as his desperate efforts to win political favour and secure a high-ranking appointment failed, Thomson was no longer able to see himself as the Aborigines' protector or saviour, and so experienced the other side of his fantasy—that of the rejected and despised outcast. As a result, he increasingly confused their plight with his own, believing *he* was the victim of 'injustice' and 'discrimination'. His own cause thereby dis-placed the Aboriginal one in his mind; time and time again he would set out to present their case, only to end up pressing his own—and in the name of 'justice'.[27]

Yet neither Thomson's increasing self-absorption nor his retreat from public life meant the political ideals he championed more than any other advocate for Aboriginal rights in the interwar and postwar decades were ignored or forgotten. After 1947 he occasionally spoke his mind on the direction of Aboriginal affairs, attacking the Commonwealth government and calling for fundamental change. These passionate outbursts made him an important figure for those critical of contemporary policy and practice. In the 1950s and 1960s his work came to be interpreted by sympathetic supporters as constituting an attack upon assimilation, and by the early 1970s his call for Aboriginal rights, especially to land, which had once seemed beyond the political pale, were increasingly moving to centre stage, though sadly Thomson did not live long enough to see this.

Some questions remain to be considered, the answers to which tell us much about Australia's racial structure, both past and present. Could anyone who was not as troubled as Thomson have been such a passionate advocate of the rights of Indigenous Australians? To what degree did his desire typify many champions of rights for Aboriginal people? And what was and is the price when non-Aboriginal advocates (can) unquestioningly assume the right to campaign on their behalf?

9

Health, hygiene and the phallic body: thoughts on psychoanalysis and history

Christopher E. Forth

Hᴵꜱᴛᴏʀʏ'ꜱ ʀᴇʟᴀᴛɪᴏɴꜱʜɪᴩ ᴛᴏ ᴩꜱʏᴄʜᴏᴀɴᴀʟʏꜱɪꜱ has been ambivalent at best, hostile at worst, and charts a tension that is itself worthy of analysis. Even cultural historians interested in intimate matters of self-identity like structures of feeling often balk at the implications of Freudian theory, expressing on the one hand admiration for the insights about the individual that it provides, while citing, as one historian claims in a recent study, 'the difficulty of finding an acceptable point of departure that does not assume too much. Psychoanalysis is both insightful and unwieldy in its assumptions about the individual.'[1] Yet employing the insights procured through psychoanalysis hardly requires a slavish adherence to every piece of Freudian doctrine, and in the past few decades scholars in a variety of fields have been inspired more by the hermeneutic promise of psychoanalysis than by its positivistic and sometimes ahistorical insistence upon the 'truth' about the unconscious.[2] For such scholars, many of whom work in or have been inspired by developments in literary criticism or cultural anthropology, psychoanalysis is one interpretive tool among many, and provides a manner of 'seeing' that illuminates developments that are not always accessible through conventional contextual methodologies. Such work approximates what Bryan Turner calls 'methodological pragmatism', a flexible stance that encourages the adjustment of one's methods in accordance with 'the nature of the problem and . . . the level of explanation which is required'.[3]

In particular psychoanalysis has the benefit of opening up more intimate dimensions to the phenomenon of 'othering' which has preoccupied so much contemporary work in the humanities and social sciences. Eric L. Santner suggests that psychoanalysis is particularly instructive in 'drawing our attention to the affective and libidinal dimensions of prejudice and has made us sensitive to the ways in which private and collective fantasies about the "other" figure in the psychosexual make-up of the human subject'.[4] The fantasmatic trappings of many stereotypes of the other thus point directly to how the self conceives of its own boundaries, of what is thought and felt to be its inside and its outside. Most importantly, psychoanalysis illustrates how the two domains are not mutually exclusive, for, as Diana Fuss indicates, 'any outside is formulated as a consequence of a lack *internal* to the system it supplements' and operates much as homosexuality does in the construction of heterosexual identity, 'as an indispensable interior exclusion —an outside which is inside interiority making the articulation of the latter possible, a transgression of the border which is necessary to constitute the border as such'.[5] Through psychoanalysis the boundaries of the ego emerge as formations intimately related to developments outside of the self, whether sociological, cultural or historical in nature.

Historians have rarely taken ego boundaries as a focal point, perhaps due to the difficulty of ascertaining such profoundly subjective borders, or perhaps due to a dearth of frank first-hand accounts of how individuals have actually experienced their embodied existence. Those who have considered such questions have necessarily had recourse to extrapolations from contemporary prescriptions about how the body ought to have been lived at any given time. Of course the gap between the normative and the experiential is an uncomfortable one, which is one reason why addressing the problem of ego boundaries means that some sort of theorisation becomes essential. This exploratory essay considers ways of extending psychoanalytic understandings of bodily boundaries to the history of the body that has emerged in the last decade or so. As a case in point, it briefly considers the experiences of Swiss philosopher Henri-Frédéric Amiel, whose twelve-volume *Journal Intime* recounts how a man's emotional investment in his sense of boundaries (and thus his identity as a man) could be closely bound up with matters of health and hygiene. This association between health and subjectivity represents an underdeveloped aspect of the history of the body, one where the judicious application of psychoanalytic concepts may prove fruitful.

Health and the bodily ego

Historians and sociologists of the body have amply demonstrated how deeply physical appearance is embedded in discourses of morality, legality and beauty, suggesting that a healthy and attractive body is, as Pierre Bourdieu observes, a most important form of social capital. A marker of youthfulness and vitality, the appearance of well-being is imbricated in matters of beauty which often promise success in social and professional situations. In addition to being potentially translatable into economic capital through the preferential treatment that often rewards physical attractiveness, health and beauty have also been viewed as forms of biological capital which promise the reproduction of desirable physicality (and its attending social benefits) across generations. The opposite effect is often the fate for those whose bodies appear unhealthy or (which amounts to the same thing) unattractive. Historically such people have found themselves located outside the sphere of the good, the true, and the beautiful by becoming associated with immorality, mendaciousness and general ugliness. All of this has implications on the level of the state itself, where the 'healthy' citizen is meant to reproduce in him/herself the integrity of the body politic.[6]

Yet how have individuals themselves wrestled with such processes? Historians say less about such issues, perhaps due to their assumption, inspired in part by the work of Michel Foucault, that social constructions operate externally through discursive frameworks that are coextensive with the body and subjectivity itself. It is not that the body does not exist, Foucault insists, but that 'the biological and the historical are not consecutive to one another'. For Foucault, a proper 'history of bodies' would consider 'the manner in which what is most material and most vital in them has been invested'.[7] Yet while we may accept Foucault's general project, must we also conclude that the inside is therefore simply a colonisation by the outside? Is there evidence that such investments could also operate from the inside out?

Contemporary feminist theory provides useful correctives to this tendency toward radical historicism, and reminds us of the *embodied* aspects of Freud's notion of the unconscious. In an often-quoted statement from *The Ego and the Id*, Freud observes that the ego is 'first and foremost a bodily ego; it is not merely a surface entity, but is itself the projection of a surface'.[8] It is this mental projection of (or libidinal investment in) the body's surface that privileges certain points or zones over others, partly through identification with the bodies of others, partly as a means of providing a sense of unity over the child's otherwise discontinuous and chaotic physical experiences. (Jacques Lacan's notion of the mirror stage vividly illustrates the specular nature of these first identifications.) It goes without saying that personal identity is impossible without some sense of subjective unity and bodily boundaries, however relative or unstable this may be; yet the observation that the bodily ego is always already implicated in sociocultural processes makes it possible to theorise shifting ego boundaries from a historical perspective. Moreover, it makes it possible to consider scenarios in which boundaries are invested differently, with greater or lesser degrees of permeability and tolerance for real or imagined intrusions from the outside.

Robert Schilder and Julia Kristeva have suggested ways of understanding the lived experience of selfhood that are useful for considering subjectivity in historical context. Schilder's work on the phantom limb phenomenon indicates how the experience of embodied selfhood proceeds through a libidinal investment in the surfaces of the body, an investment that persists despite the loss of certain bodily parts. Similarly, Kristeva employs the idea of abjection to demonstrate how the experience of bodily cohesion depends upon expelling from one's identity corporeal substances that are disavowed as elements of the self, thus revealing how one's body image rests on a continual abjection of substances like dirt, faeces, blood, and mucus. As a process that requires continual repetition, abjection underlies the fantasmatic nature of the self, whereby, as Judith Butler argues, 'the subject is constituted through the force of exclusion and abjection, one which produces a constitutive outside to the subject, an abjected outside which is, after all, "inside" the subject as its own founding repudiation'.[9]

Although abjection seems to be a virtually universal and unavoidable aspect of any coherent sense of identity, it operates differently across gender lines. Kristeva and Mary Douglas point to the gender dynamic that seems inherent in abjection by emphasising how closely women are associated, through sexuality and menstruation, with filth and dirt, and in a sense come to embody the abject itself. Grosz quite rightly claims that in the Western world women's bodies have been understood in terms of formlessness, flow and viscosity; through their capacity for menstruation and sexual penetration 'women's corporeality is inscribed as a mode of seepage'.[10] As Grosz sees it, 'the attribution of a phallic or castrated status to sexually differentiated bodies is an internal condition of the ways those bodies are lived and given meaning right from the start (with or without the child's knowledge or compliance)'.[11] If women are thus so closely implicated in the collapse of boundaries, then a sensible next step would be to investigate the foundations of masculine identity as pertaining to that group historically considered more capable of sustaining a cohesive and impermeable sense of self. In other words, if the bodies of women have frequently been seen (and lived) as 'leaky' or 'castrated' in one way or another, it is worth considering what it means for a male to experience his body as 'phallic'.[12]

There is ample evidence that the development of the modern notion of the self is predicated on ideals of autonomy, rectitude and closure which are decidedly phallic in nature. Many historians agree that the Western conception of the atomised, self-contained and autonomous male self is of fairly recent vintage, and that it emerged in the fifteenth and sixteenth centuries against the backdrop of a collapsing feudal system, a new scientific and artistic focus on the human as both the object and subject of science and culture, free enterprise, a rising bourgeoisie, and a Protestant focus on freedom of religious conviction. Less recognised by historians is the fact that this transformation also entailed a new mode of embodiment, a way of living the new-found autonomy and inwardness of the self on a day-to-day basis. Some scholars have provided useful ways of conceptualising this shift in bodily styles. In his study of the popular sensibilities that circulated in the bawdy works of François Rabelais, for example, Mikhail Bakhtin demonstrates how the grotesque body of premodern Europe provoked an ambivalence about bodily functions that was never manifested as a simple rejection. Indeed, the grotesque body was treated as unfinished and as always overflowing its boundaries, thus continually integrating the 'higher' functions with the 'lower material bodily strata' where digestive, excretory, sexual and reproductive functions reside. In its focus on liminal physical functions like eating, drinking, excretion, copulation, pregnancy, dismemberment and being devoured by another, the grotesque body reveals the essentially porous nature of the body in its openness towards the world. 'Contrary to modern canons, the grotesque body is not separated from the rest of the world. It is not a closed, completed unit; it is unfinished, outgrows itself, transgresses its own limits.'[13]

The cultivation of a more bounded sense of self entailed a reworking of this older conception of the body, a process shaped by the rise of the bourgeoisie and a reorientation of gender roles. Bakhtin suggests that it called for a new body marked by an inner hierarchy wherein the 'lower' sexual and excretory functions were strictly separated from 'higher'. Peter Stallybrass and Allon White have extended this idea into the modern period to show that this topography was in part constructed through hygienic conceptions of the personal body and the body politic where, in addition to the boundary between inside and outside, a

> vertical axis of the bourgeois body is primarily emphasised in the *education* of the child: as s/he grows up/is cleaned up, the lower bodily stratum is regulated or denied, as far as possible, by the correct posture ('stand up straight', 'don't squat', 'don't kneel on all fours'—the postures of servants and savages), and by the censoring of lower 'bodily' references along with bodily wastes.

The 'lower' bodily zone thus became likened to

> the *city's* 'low'—the slum, the rag-picker, the prostitute, the sewer—the 'dirt' which is 'down there'. In other words, the axis of the body is transcoded through the axis of the city, and whilst the bodily low is 'forgotten', the city's low becomes a site of obsessive preoccupation, a preoccupation which is itself intimately conceptualised in terms of discourses of the body.[14]

In other words, attention to hygiene and general health were, and continue to be, essential to the maintenance of the bourgeois body as 'a strictly completed, finished product' where all 'signs of its unfinished character, of its growth and proliferation were eliminated'.[15]

New hygienic knowledge was in fact abetted by these new attitudes. As Norbert Elias has demonstrated, the shifts in sensibility about bodily functions that one observes in sixteenth-century etiquette manuals preceded any new scientific developments, suggesting that a process of social and psychic distancing was already underway without any need for a scientific rationale. In a sense Elias's history of manners is an attempt, if not to describe precisely the location of ego boundaries, then to demonstrate how the prescriptions provided by etiquette manuals helped to instil in young males a sense of bodily boundedness by fostering disgust at activities and substances that had hitherto not been encoded as abject. In experiential terms the lived body that Elias observes certainly appears to have been more closed—and closed off—than previous ones, and serves as a useful example of how the boundary formation that would characterise the new sense of self was slowly being created. What Elias describes as the boundaries being sketched around and within the sixteenth-century bodies emerge as aspects of a libidinal investment in the ideal of bodily closure based more on personal and collective fantasy than on medical fact.[16]

As the male body was taken as the standard of good health, it is easy to see how its phallic qualities could be affirmed through hygiene. Good health was often described as a suit of armour that insulated one from pathogens and other external physical threats, thus maximising man's ability to exercise willpower and initiative. In so far as good health signified ethical rectitude and the maintenance of bodily order, hygienic precepts were moral injunctions that allowed for resistance to less tangible influences, particularly the sensual seductions often encountered in urban centres. As we will see in the case of Amiel, the libidinal investment in the body's surface was predicated to a significant degree on the presumed relationship between subjective integrity and physical soundness. Amiel's failure to achieve physical health was correspondingly experienced as a rupture of ego boundaries, resulting in a crisis of manhood and subjectivity generally.

Henri-Frédéric Amiel: 'to be a man just once before death'

The twelve-volume *Journal Intime* of the Swiss philosopher Henri-Frédéric Amiel (1821–81) presents an astonishingly frank account of one man's personal struggle to achieve what he considered to be an adequate embodiment of normative manhood, a gender identity frustrated as much by physical weakness as by his problematic status as a bachelor and a sedentary intellectual. Written over the course of thirty years with the eventual aim of publication, the *Journal Intime* records Amiel's incessant self-examination, what he called 'a monomania of circumspection' where his imperious and judgmental 'I' would often submit a less-than-ideal 'you' to the most intimate and merciless criticism.[17] Most importantly, Amiel's confessions suggest how during the nineteenth century conventional forms of masculinity depended upon moral and physical integrity that rendered the self *phallic* (firm, self-contained, upright, masterful) in its relationship with external influences. In both physical and moral terms, much of Amiel's adult life was lived in accordance with Rousseau's injunction that one should 'be a man just once before death', thus indicating the rather elusive character of normative gender roles. Given the sheer volume of writing that Amiel devoted to recounting his daily experiences and the preliminary stage of my own investigations, the discussion that follows is necessarily tentative and speculative, and is concerned primarily with marking areas where a fruitful dialogue between history and psychoanalysis could take place.

Like many other bourgeois individuals, Amiel paid particular attention to hygiene as a means of warding off illness and rendering his body fit. Washing his body daily 'from the soles of his feet to the roots of his hair' had become for him 'a voluptuous act, even a need. This friction awakens and refines, tones and renders the body supple.' Catching sight of his naked body in the mirror also offered a rare opportunity for narcissistic investment in his body image, where 'innocent indifference replaced the furtive shame at seeing myself without clothes'. Posing before the mirror revealed many things to him: 'first of all, my body is well built and well shaped, all the lines are correct, the overall design is exquisite and virile, the shape of the torso and shoulders [is] irreproachable'. Amiel's pleasure at these impressions was clear and they filled him with pride: 'I felt as if I were in a Spartan gymnasium'.[18] Such practices seemed to harmonise Amiel's body image with his kinaesthetic impressions, producing in him the sensation of resilience and 'elasticity' that was synonymous with physical well-being and which allowed him to confront and withstand daily worries without being overwhelmed by them. 'Health is elasticity', he once declared, and it implied 'independence of the climate and of the outside world'.[19]

The hygienic practices that aimed at producing, recovering, or sustaining health were 'the art of extracting from the organism all the energy and health it is capable of supplying', and thus providing a foundation of physical force that would allow him to remain cohesive as a man. As a young man Amiel summarised the overall aims of his hygienic practices: '*to render nervous and intellectual life as energetic, active, elastic, and obedient as possible*—to augment my capacity for work without surpassing my own forces.—To train myself in vigorous effort and prolonged effort: with the leap of a tiger and the patience of a mole [emphasis in original].'[20] The value of clean air and water, particularly fresh, running water, was central to the hydrotherapeutic regimen that Amiel followed, and was essential to establishing elasticity: 'Free air caresses the skin; spring water renders the same service to the digestive tract. It is only through the double ablution of our accessible surface that we recover elasticity.'[21] In addition to water-based therapies, gymnastics too was on Amiel's list of practices that promised to produce 'vigour and elasticity'.[22]

The pleasure that Amiel took in his own physicality was nevertheless limited and fleeting, and most of his subsequent references to his body reveal profound self-consciousness and shame. Whatever fantasies Amiel had about approximating ideal manhood were undermined by his own somatic experiences. As a more or less sedentary academic with a propensity toward shyness, Amiel felt alienated from the overtly physical ideal that has been undergirded in the West by what Michael Nerlich terms the 'ideology of adventure', a 'systematic glorification of the (knightly, then bourgeois) adventurer as the most developed and important human being'.[23] When writing in the guise of an imperious 'I', Amiel found his state of existence to be quite pathetic. Reflecting upon his aversion to wild animals, for instance, his 'I' was without mercy. 'Man should be more brutal and coarse than that . . . Man should know how to eviscerate and kill . . . What you lack is a bit of ferocity; having neither gone hunting or camping, you are decidedly too soft; you are too much of a woman.'[24] He agreed with the advice of a friend about how to improve his abject condition:

> I should make my delicateness, my character and my style a bit more *brutal*, to dip my feet in the river Styx for a little while, that is to say to *masculinise* myself, and to virilise myself, to marshal [*aguerrir*] my courage, to tighten my will, that is to say, to become someone and something [emphasis in original].[25]

Amiel's inability to approximate the warrior ethos was compounded by the health problems that, despite his hygienic efforts, he repeatedly described in his journal. Here he equated manliness with physical robustness in terms of the capacity for resistance that was lacking in more refined social circles:

> True health means indifference to atmospheric conditions, because it creates its own atmosphere. The stronger one is, the less sensitive he is to all that torments, agitates, worries and upsets worldly people. Robustness is a suit of armour and consequently a source of freedom. Vulnerability is a hard servitude. *Vae debilibus!* Woe to the weaklings![26]

The 'armour' to which he sometimes referred also connoted emotional hardness, which explains why allowing himself to experience emotions in a 'feminine' manner necessarily compromised this sense of protection. When corresponding with two female friends in 1855, for example, he reported feeling 'invaded' by the softness of tender feelings that threatened to undermine him. 'The siren of sympathies laced enervating incantations within me ... I had the need to love and to be loved, and a love-potion circulated in my veins. My armour was unbuckled, I was disarmed and nearly vanquished.' This moment of weakness was for Amiel the 'anti-heroic state, the moment when man is most vulnerable to the arrows of voluptuousness'.[27]

Self-mastery and health were thus the elusive aims of Amiel's adult life. 'What saddens me is having only rarely experienced the feeling of physical well-being and health.'[28] 'And what is health?' he reflected again in 1868: 'The overabundance of force, the opulence of life'.[29] Physical health also meant being insulated from external stimuli of every sort, for in 'an enervated state all spontaneity is diminished and dependence on outside influences increases'.[30] On the one hand this could mean susceptibility to changes in the weather,[31] but it could also suggest an insulation against social conditions that could also affect one's sense of autonomy. Here Amiel chastised himself for being emotionally porous, for being 'much too impressionable, and sympathetically infectible, I feel exhausted, weakened, depressed by contact with frail and broken down people [*les êtres caduques*]. Inversely, proximity to healthy people resuscitates me and likable company electrifies me.' This 'involuntary imitation' may have been useful intellectually, he confessed, but it took him far from the masculine ideal to which he aspired: 'it is fatal for action ... What is lacking in me, I know it well, is brutality, which imposes itself on the outside world and dominates other wills'.[32] Being susceptible to the influence of others prompted Amiel to reflect upon the damage he was doing to himself by frequenting the company of women. 'In the sweetness of feminine society', he wrote, 'one feminises and softens oneself ...' Even as a young man he compared himself unfavourably to men with 'more vigour, but less delicacy; more muscles, fewer nerves'.[33]

Nervous weakness, or enervation, represented for Amiel a source of constant weakness and anxiety, and was the source of his emotional frailty. 'When I am in an enervated state, as I have been lately', he wrote in 1872, 'I experience imagined sicknesses or miseries with as much intensity as if they were real.—My weakness makes me realise that *virtue* is a form of courage, a force, a virility; and that the weak man ceases to be a man'.[34] The kind of enervation wrought through masturbation and nocturnal emissions was central to Amiel's health concerns, and remained his most persistent complaint well into old age. So common were his guilty expenditures that in his diary he resorted to the abbreviation 'ps' (*perte séminale*) to record these scourges. As was the case with many men, Amiel experienced vividly most of the symptoms the doctors had led him to expect: headaches, palpitations, memory problems and nervousness. Unconsciousness was tantamount to an unbuckling of Amiel's armour, which is why erotic dreams were for him another instance of a collapse of boundaries, a crisis of integrity that was as much moral as it was physical. 'What a useless breach!' he once complained after a wet dream.[35]

Yet semen loss was not the only source of Amiel's enervation, for the medical wisdom of the day also held that nervous energy was just as easily depleted through excessive mental labour: in other words, the man of letters who read too much was often likened to a masturbator who cavalierly squandered his energy.[36] The act of writing in his diary was for Amiel but one more example of how he continually depleted himself, wasting his virility on unproductive activities that he once deplored as 'logo-diarrhea':[37]

> The habit of dispensing my sentiments, my chagrins or my resolutions in words, in solitary monologues, has contributed to that. This Journal is a release-valve [*un exutoire*]; my virility evaporates in the sweat of ink . . . I have often thought that the redaction of these pages was a replacement for life, a variety of onanism.[38]

As a substitute for true action, this endless inner scrutiny 'emasculated me', and constituted a 'eunuchism renewed on a daily basis, like castration through personal critique'.[39] If he were ever to marry, he speculated, then his wife would become a substitute for his daily scribbles, 'a living journal, a confessional, a second conscience, a rebuilding of what the world destroys in us'.[40] Without such a living presence Amiel was thrown back on the solitary musings that ultimately weakened him: 'revery emasculates like opium . . . Far from being instinctive, the defence of your integrity, of your personal existence, is a recurring problem . . . Solitude. Revery (mental onanism). Sterility. Suicide, all of these form a series'.[41]

For years Amiel was haunted by the spectre of this physical depletion, which he envisioned as a weakening or 'castration' of a body that he had come to see as ideally phallic: 'Enervation resembles castration. It diminishes one's being. One is no longer anything but a half-man'.[42] Manhood appears here as a quality dispersed throughout the body and manifested in energy, willpower and force, which is why the diminishment of these traits could appear as a form of emasculation. His weakness and indecision often made him feel like 'a man on retreat, on holiday' who has begged off all responsibility in exchange for peace and quiet. 'This great lassitude that precedes all effort has nothing heroic or interesting about it; it is despair or cowardice or premature old age.' Here too his physical and mental weaknesses reflected sadly on the state of his body as a failed phallus, for such 'wise timidity makes a species of eunuchs . . . I am entirely passive, drifting, indifferent . . .'[43] To be so bereft of spontaneity and vitality was no longer to be a man; rather, such apathy represented 'a state of sterility, of eunuchism, of impotence. In fact, it is a sort of intermittent castration'.[44]

The language Amiel used to describe the effects of these castrations on his sense of self conveyed a clear impression of fluidity and the dissolution of manhood, the loss of his 'individual cohesion'.[45] The aging Amiel regretted that he was falling into

> the category of weakened men. I am not ill, but all my vitality is diminished. I am more than delicate, I am susceptible, impressionable, easily tired, languishing, enervated . . . The happiness of inhabiting a ready, docile and robust body, where the mind functions with ease, is this happiness thus lost for me?

Weaklings such as he

> tend to come apart [*se déagréger*]. Liquefaction is the beginning of destruction since it undoes structure . . . Individuality rests on character, which is the result of will, which is a force. An individuality without force is a crystal that dissolves in a bath, a cloud that is reabsorbed into the atmosphere, it is something that dies and is effaced.[46]

Amiel's disturbing sensation of collapse was intimately related to obsessions about his flagging physical health. Arguing against conventional notions of bodily integrity as being synonymous with an unchanging state of health and soundness, Gail Weiss posits a more dynamic conception in which 'bodily integrity is *created* through developing a greater sensitivity to one's bodily changes, capacities, movements, and gestures . . . [it is] the denial of the co-existence of disparate sensations and movements that threatens the consistency of bodily experience'.[47] Amiel's case seems to illustrate Weiss's point, where his tendency to glorify the hardness and integrity manifested by other men only exacerbated his own sense of failure and effeminacy.

To take Amiel as an exemplar of nineteenth-century bourgeois manhood would of course be an exaggeration, for his obsessions about health and manhood were no doubt somewhat unique. Nevertheless his remarks are in keeping with the medical literature of his day, and provide a useful illustration of how physical integrity could be so emotionally invested as to become virtually synonymous with selfhood (and how its absence could signify the draining or castration of a body that was ideally replete, masterful, and impermeable). Traditional historiography is of little use when dealing with cases such as Amiel's, and even the cultural historian would require more sophisticated tools when trying to analyse the relationship between hygiene and selfhood. Although further work is required on Amiel, it is evident that psychoanalysis provides indispensable tools for any historian hoping to make sense of this compelling case.

III

The psyche of national identities

10

Identity: history, the nation and the self

Notes on a conceptual itinerary, 1967–2001

Miriam Dixson

THIS CHAPTER REFLECTS on a conceptual itinerary which I have pursued since 1967. Focused on Australia as part of the West, that itinerary first drew on Danish-American psychoanalyst Erik Erikson, the so-called architect of identity. It was in the 1960s that Erikson ignited my interest in the relation between national identity, historical change and the work of the ego.

In the late 1970s, under the influences of feminism and an increasing recognition of the split nature of the self, I began to engage with the ideas of the British Object Relations School and of Melanie Klein in particular. In object-relations theory inner objects are unconscious representations of relationships, primarily concerning parents and other significant early figures. Initially my engagement with object relations was sparked by Klein's relevance to feminist theory as demonstrated in Dorothy Dinnerstein's book *The Mermaid and the Minotaur*. (More later about Dinnerstein.) But Klein ranged far beyond feminist issues: her underlying problematic was the divided modern to late-modern self in its struggle towards a workable, 'good-enough' integration. In keeping with the British psychoanalytic object-relations tradition, Klein's recurrent themes concern the two most basic characteristics of the self: on the one hand, the deeply split nature of the self, and on the other, its inherent thrust toward imperfect but workable integration. For Klein, 'development is essentially a move from fragmentation to integration'.[1] We can see her as a postmodernist who rejected the nihilist refusal of postmodernism to recognise as central to our being the self's pilgrimage towards workable integration. By the late 1980s, I remained puzzled and intrigued as to how national identity was laid down and how it persisted. For this I turned finally to the ideas of Cornelius Castoriadis. A former Greek insurgent, Trotskyist and more recently psychoanalyst, Castoriadis was also the philosopher of the social imaginary.

Closer to its heart than many would wish, today's Australian identity still carries the marks of yesterday's British connection. For all its rich current ethnic diversity, Australian identity remains shot through with the habits of the heart, the anthropological ways, of its anchoring Anglo-Celtic core. On this, coherence and stability for our multicultural democracy might continue to depend for some transitional years. Basic institutions, population statistics, political custom, values and family ties go far to explain why Anglo-Celtic (henceforth Anglo) ways have proved so enduring in Australia. But there is also the social imaginary.

Philosopher Paul Ricoeur defines the social imaginary as 'an opaque kernel' 'beyond or beneath the self-understanding of a society'. For any given society, the social imaginary is the 'foundational mytho-poetic nucleus', a nucleus 'constitutive of a culture before it can be expressed and reflected in specific representations or ideas'.[2] Later we examine the social imaginary as envisaged by Castoriadis, but here we merely note a strong correspondence between the social imaginary as this country's 'foundational mytho-poetic nucleus' and the mental universe of early Anglo Australia.

Drawing on Erikson, Klein and Castoriadis to explore identity, my conceptual itinerary is best expressed in two books: *The Real Matilda: Women and Identity in Australia, 1788 to the Present* (in its four editions from 1976 to 1999); and *The Imaginary Australian: Anglo-Celts and Identity—1788 to the Present* (1999).[3]

Erik Erikson, who died in 1994, was a proponent of what came to be called 'ego psychoanalysis'. (Though deeply tied to the unconscious, the ego is the mental agent closest to 'reality'.) Erikson was German-born of Danish-Jewish parents. Encountering Freud's Vienna Circle in the 1920s, analysed by Anna Freud and drawn to her pioneering work on child analysis, Erikson and his young family fled in 1933 from Nazism to the United States. He became Boston's first child psychoanalyst. As a young man riven with aching inner conflict—'on the border between neurosis and psychosis' and in his own view 'probably close to psychosis'[4]—Erikson would go on to establish 'identity' as a defining concept for our times.

Working with anthropologists, sociologists and historians, Erikson developed a theory about the stages of the life cycle. During each stage, the ego synthesised and resynthesised inner (psychic) and outer (social-historical) worlds around conflicting basic attitudes. (The adolescent stage has entered our vocabulary as the 'identity crisis'.) The outcome of each

engagement between conflicting basic attitudes builds on the results of preceding engagements, but in each new stage insight can creatively recast
aspects of antecedent encounters. Broadly congruent with bodily development, the psyche's unfolding struggles are essentially relational and moral
in character: this is what most clearly aligns Erikson with British object-
relations analysts like Klein and Donald Winnicott.[5] The stages of ego conflict begin in infancy with the clash of 'trust versus mistrust' and end in old
age with that of 'integrity versus despair'.[6]

Grounded strongly in a sense of history, Erikson's work targeted the
register of social change within the psyche, using terms which included
class, gender, race, religious and national identifications. To be sure, like so
many analysts who fled Hitler to America, Erikson lost a good deal of the
subversive, nocturnal vision shared by early Freudians. Thus while savaging
the destructive aspects of global and American corporatism, Erikson over
emphasised the ego's adaptiveness and creativity. Bland at its worst, this
over emphasis risked underplaying both the self's inner contradictions and
the malevolent sides of late capitalism. Yet at its best, as with Castoriadis,
Erikson's work registered the fact that this chaotic, violent era contains the
most breathtaking creative potential.

Erikson holds special interest for the Australian historian of identity. For
Erikson, the post-sixteenth-century settler-capitalist lands of Europe (such
as Australia) are societies under the rule of the brother rather than the
father. Central to authority as much as to gender, this shift within male domination set a vital parameter for my understanding of women and identity
and of Australian identity as a whole. From faint beginnings in seventeenth-
century Europe, the never-to-be-total shift from fatherly (patriarchal) to
brotherly (fratriarchal) male domination quickly moved to centre stage in
frontier capitalist-settler nations. (After the mid-twentieth century we see
its global spread.) Entailing an increasingly tenuous sense of male and of
social authority, this generational shift in male domination offered women
astonishing new possibilities.

In 1964 Harvard political philosopher Louis Hartz published *The
Founding of New Societies*. The book was a study of what he called 'fragment'
societies—America, Canada, Australia and others—which were spun off
Europe after the sixteenth century. Hartz argued that the old-world political structures of founding inhabitants came to be 'formative' for the politics
of each new-world 'fragment' society. Thus America became a middle-class
'liberal polity' and Australia a working-class 'radical-democratic' polity.[7]
But Hartz gave us no adequate explanation of *how* his founding political
configurations (designed to be richly suggestive rather than pedantically
accurate) were able to persist over time. However, in effectively expanding
Hartz's basic approach beyond politics, Erikson had offered what we can see

as an explanation for such persistence. Beginnings and early experiences, Erikson thought, were formative not merely, as Hartz believed, for political structures but for society across the board. They were formative in respect of the fragment society's sense of authority, of sex role, of work patterns and so on. Even while cleaving close to kin and tradition, when migrants arrived in a new land, in the cause of survival they also adapted to the wider mores already present, adapted to what already worked and so made possible their ongoing social existence. But how were the key social attitudes and values underwriting such adaptation actually handed down? Erikson held that they were transmitted during the process of socialisation, beginning with the mother–baby relation and its powerful unconscious (thus preverbal) component. However, as we see later, for Castoriadis there is more to culture transmission than socialisation.

Historians often tell us that the past lives on in the present. For example, in his classic 1930 book *Australia*, Keith Hancock (this country's Tocqueville) suspected that 'there has come down to us, by subtle hidden channels, a vague unmeasured inheritance from those early days'.[8] Here Hancock refers to the convict inheritance. (For example, Australians, he thought, viewed the state as a 'milch cow', and for him this view was part of the convict inheritance.) But historians rarely ask the question of *how* such legacies come down to us over the generations.

Before suggesting a further answer to this question, we consider some other legacies which, like convictism, threw long shadows forward to the future. In the case of colonial Australia, one central legacy concerned 'respectability'. Through its ability to promote rebellion as much as conformity, respectability was a cultural leitmotif in colonial Australia and throughout the West. British imperial opinion derogated Australians as lamentably deficient in respectability; not only were they colonial, they were convict-colonial. The British view evoked strong ego defenses in our hegemonic classes. Importantly for this reason, Australian elites, along with all who internalised dominant imperial prescription, along with all who aspired to the bourgeois condition of respectability, experienced a disabling sense of illegitimacy. Australian defenses against this sense of illegitimacy targeted women and their potential for autonomy. Fastening on the female convict as the paramount symbol of female *un*respectability, respectability for colonial women defensively ballooned into ultrarespectability and ultra-domesticity. For a long time, such defenses would sap women's energies, especially their political and intellectual energies.[9]

This extremely brief excursus on colonial legacies now turns to religion. From as early as the sixteenth century, religion—its nature, its strengths and weaknesses—played a huge part in shaping national identity (the old, established nations of Europe have very early origins[10]). If one compares the religious dimension of life in nineteenth-century England, America and Australia, it is clear that during Australia's formative moments, the focus on underlying ideological matters like salvation was much less sharp than in England or the United States. Thus issues of observance and, later, social reform trumped those of transcendence. This helps explain why, in general, Anglo Australians tend to deal with any form of ideology at its surface levels. Finally, to the extent that effectively atheist historians have tended to set its terms, national identity discourse skirts the religious dimension of identity and deals awkwardly with much of the whole symbolic realm.

The flavour of Australian colonial living was often harsh, often ugly and cruel, though perhaps not more than that of comparable settler countries. However from the start, everyday life (the lifeworld) also knew broad-ranging decency, dogged courage, ready kindness and fellowship. As to Erikson's (and our) crucial identity issue of ego autonomy, several conflicting concerns vie for attention. Restricting autonomy—here there are contrasts with early America—was the convict state and the formative cultural weight of the so-called convict churches, the Anglican and Catholic. But from the start—here there are parallels with America—important countervailing forces made themselves felt. Even if scarred by the centralism of the founding convict state, Australia's structuring political and social institutions were cut from British prototypes at a moment when these were the most representative in the history of civilisation. At the time most human societies were characterised by 'the rule of one' (as Montesquieu put it), and in and of themselves, representative institutions ('the rule of several') encouraged autonomy. But autonomy was greatly strengthened where, in the context of a stable, constitutionally based state, a robust civil society emerged. As Marx (no lover of British institutions) pointed out, in respect of such a civil society, England led the world. Despite their strong central state, from the 1790s Anglo Australians were the antipodean bearers of civil society and its defining voluntary, non-hierarchical (but not always morally virtuous) associational mode. Thus from Australia's formative years, a centralised government and an ineffective local authority were to a degree offset—we should not exaggerate the degree—by the activism and thrust to ego autonomy inherent in civil society.

These, then, were some of the influences which, in a contradictory mix, would form enduring patterns in Australia's Anglo culture. Resilience, egalitarianism and fairness where non-indigenous Australians were concerned —such qualities put down sturdy roots. But in a convict-frontier situation, the heart was so often lacerated. Scars sustained by Anglo culture in early encounters with exile and loneliness, with Indigenous Australians, with a bitterly alien environment, found representation in the social imaginary itself. Massive denial alone enabled Anglo culture to face the life and death tasks of pioneering. So the habit, the mechanism, of denial—including of course emotional denial—also found their imaginary representation. Thus as Erikson shows in the case of frontier Anglo America, the ego defended against formative cultural wounds in part by denying or forcefully restricting emotion, and to an extent which greatly diminished the possibilities of relationship.

At the beginning of the twenty-first century, Anglo identity still harbours aspects of colonial experience which time has sedimented into the culture. At bone level, there remains an assumption of equality by ordinary people. Largely the outcome of colonial Australian and earlier European struggles over rights and representative institutions (the outcome too of *experiencing* those institutions), this assumption owes much to the common people, to their sacrifices and passionate activism. Take the eighteenth-century British radical religious and proto-trade-union story; take the struggles of the 1640 English Civil War. We could go back much earlier.

Given Australia's formative and traumatic geographical separation from kin communities, and given the lifeworld distortions inherent in convictism as founding institution, racist tendencies in Anglo Australia were at least as strong as those of comparable societies. (Any reliable verdict on this must await a careful comparative perspective lacking in most relevant research.) Old-identity Anglo qualities also include an unusually strong version of male bonding known as mateship. This helped produce what, measured against comparable and cousin societies, was in many ways an aridly masculine culture. But mateship has its blessings too. In the early twenty-first century, state and market incursions into the family and thus into parenting work alongside global corporatism to shred the social texture which ultimately sustains democracy. (This is the most fateful of the down sides which accompany the breathtaking promise of globalisation.) Thus today the solidarities of Anglo mateship help offset a perilous social fracturing.

In 1976 in *The Real Matilda* I argued that Anglo-Australian culture at that time was characterised by a stronger sexism and a greater gender gulf than existed in comparable societies. Today this is far less, if at all, true, even if only because of the massive historical crisis in male work, parenting and cultural authority. *The Real Matilda* also drew attention to the fact that, in comparative context, women's public profile was unusually modest. Today second-wave feminism together with that massive male identity crisis have removed this gender characteristic as a defining Anglo-Australian pattern.

Old-identity Anglo-Australian qualities today further include a complacent yet muscular anti-intellectualism (to be sure, in this Australia is scarcely alone). Historically the mind at its less-than-practical levels has been one of our species' highest humanising features, cutting life-giving swathes into ancient jungles of ignorance and violence. Though rarely articulated, at some level of being this is very widely—perhaps almost universally—sensed. Australian anti-intellectualism, meekly endured because deeply internalised by intellectuals (*'I'm* not an intellectual—just a novelist, an editor, an academic, just doing my job'[11]), goes unremarked where not haughtily denied. But in fact the mind at its less-than-practical levels is deemed elite. Treated as the tallest of Tall Poppies, it sparks what is at source an anti-imperial defensiveness which resonates with bitter colonial memories. In all, the mind at its less-than-practical levels bows under the yoke of a relentless curdled envy. Yet just as insistently, colonial experience also threw up positive energies. Modestly offsetting the globalist fracturing of social fabric, Anglo culture (at least at its less elevated social levels) still retains something of a less-than-puritan colonial dedication to the work ethic. And in the teeth of hypercompetitive violence, Anglo Australia also maintains a surprising degree of its old commitment to fairness.

Beyond all this, for some, Anglo identity is lived most acutely on the pulses. Before I *understand* my own sense of Anglo identity through the lens of history, I *feel* it (as critic and lover, as friend not flatterer) in terms of shared creaturely qualities. Is the social imaginary experienced above all as a common creatureliness? In 1991 historian Manning Clark might have been giving cerebral expression to a visceral sense about this: 'I think it is possible to identify an Australian ... I think you identify him [*sic*] by the way he talks, even by the way he walks and his face'.[12]

So far this retrospective on my use of identity theory over some three decades has underlined Erik Erikson, whose theory was cut basically from classical Freud. Focused on the father, this gave women a derivative place. But Melanie Klein, to whom my identity concerns shifted after 1978, moved the mother to centre stage. In theorising the psychic roots of male dominance, Dorothy Dinnerstein, the so-called mothering feminist theorist who did most to shape my approach to feminism, drew centrally on Klein's seminal concepts of splitting and integration.

Dinnerstein's book *The Mermaid and the Minotaur* explored the unconscious sources of patriarchal gender with poetic directness and superb intellectual force.[13] She proposes that the roots of patriarchy lie in the immense power which the infant (wildly misreading the 'real' social situation), unconsciously senses is held by the early mother: women's perceived *power* in the nursery provides the key to women's *powerlessness* in society. Dinnerstein argues that one pan-human cultural custom underpins this power issue: women's near monopoly of early child-rearing. That near monopoly results in an unconscious gender script which she believed was basic to male domination, seen as essentially transhistorical and cross-cultural.

Feeling itself merged with, swamped by, the early mother, the infant is compelled to separate from her. Dinnerstein's theory considers the implications for adult sex roles of unconscious scripts written by the very young child in its fateful struggle towards separation and individuation. The infant unconsciously experiences the mother in terms of a richly ambivalent (adored, yet loathed because feared), high-octane and arbitrary power. That power is felt as both enthralling and monstrous, and the child must separate from its merger with the mother who wields it. What to do? This is where Dinnerstein, inspired by Klein, introduces the potent yet primitive and facile psychic mechanism of splitting. We could say that the central evolutionary function of splitting has now been overtaken because our capacities for a more mature, or 'integrated', mode of thinking have become so great. Yet the reality is that splitting remains extravagantly overprivileged. This, Dinnerstein insists, is because the patriarchal gender script continues to deploy it centrally in the process of separation.

Better known and later to emerge in the child than splitting, Freud's concept of repression applies to isolated impulses, wishes, or memories. Splitting has wider and deeper implications, for it draws together a whole cluster of elements to form a complex mental creation or creations.[14] Once split off, these are entirely dissociated from consciousness and hence basically unavailable as constructive resources for the developing self. If persisting and extensive, on both social and personal levels splitting makes for a subjectivity which, in widely varying ways, exhibit degrees of impoverishment. Early feminist theorists rightly suspected that sexism and racism employ splitting (along with projection) to expel the Other from a shared humanity. Dinnerstein, trained as a cognitive psychologist, agrees but goes further: by unduly privileging splitting, by fatefully discouraging fuller use of the more mature mechanism of 'integration', patriarchy, she contends, uses its gender script to hold back human development.

This is how. In order to move beyond its initial merged-with-the-mother state, in order to begin the process of separation, the infant *splits* its ambivalent, hugely inflated image of the mother into an all-Good mother and an all-Bad mother. As Klein put it in 1935, when through splitting 'the ego endeavours to keep the good apart from the bad', 'the result is a conception of extremely bad and extremely perfect objects'.[15] The infant then projects the mother's extremely perfect or all-Good side onto the father. (Depending on culture and political tradition, this can leave the mother so excessively 'Bad' as to facilitate a Talibanesque-treatment.) When the child escapes from (what it unconsciously feels to be) the rampant, arbitrary power of the early mother into the arms of the father, the child is committing itself to patriarchy, the seemingly more benign rule of the father. But, says Dinnerstein, if father and mother took an equal share in child-rearing from early infancy, the child would be compelled to employ the integrating card more and the splitting card less. No more ogress mother and no more godlike father. Mother and father would each appear to the child as flawed fellow beings, neither perfect nor monstrous. Even more important for Dinnerstein, the same move demotes splitting and promotes integration for *the whole mental repertoire of our species*.

Dinnerstein's culturalist theory of patriarchy is persuasive, indeed compelling. In locating patriarchy and its gender script close to the heart of humankind's existential dilemmas, she chooses a context which gives feminism its most ambitious claim, one surpassing even equality. Dinnerstein also proposes that women both resist and collude with a patriarchy which now, she argues, retards humankind's emotional, moral and cognitive growth. At the most basic level (there are so many others), patriarchy does this by overprivileging splitting to the detriment of integration. Dinnerstein's choice of territory seems right: the early mother–infant relation, a father starting to become 'vivid' for a child shaping gender as it engages with the fateful task of separation. But despite remarkable change in the parenting commitments of Western fathers, Dinnerstein has clearly misread something her solution mandates: the willingness of either parent to *radically* redraw the ancient parental division of labour. Suggesting a critical weakness in her approach, Dinnerstein fatally underestimates the strength of the bond between infant and mother.

Remaining with me after thirty years are two questions. With its often-enchanting, often-infuriating but stubbornly enduring ways of differentiating self and other, how is national identity initially laid down? And how does it persist over long stretches of time? For answers I turned to the social philosopher and psychoanalyst Cornelius Castoriadis, arguably 'the most formidably brilliant theorist of the complex relations between the individual and society' in postwar Europe.[16] For the light they throw on these questions, I now consider Castoriadis's concepts of the social imaginary, the 'imaginary institution of society', and the 'project of autonomy'.

We saw that for Erik Erikson, early national qualities persist through continuities handed down in the socialisation process, in which he underlines mother–baby communication and its potent unconscious component. There is a strong case for Erikson's view, but Castoriadis's social imaginary opens the way to a more complex account of cultural transmission. It suggests that even as the family and later institutions socialise the child, significant elements of continuity may always-already be present as part of a strange domain of cultural meaning beyond accepted understandings of socialisation. This is the domain of the social imaginary.[17]

The imagination is known to psychoanalysis and philosophy (Aristotle, Spinoza, Kant) alike.[18] But it is Castoriadis alone who draws on both to develop a theory explicitly around the *creativity* of the imagination: around its capacity to bring into being the non-existent. (Freud and Klein referred to unconscious fantasies without focusing on this capacity.) For Castoriadis, the radical imagination in *individual* subjectivity, morally neither positive nor negative but thoroughly ambivalent, consists of intrapsychically generated representations. In its parallel but separate function in *social* life, the social imaginary includes institutions, language and history.[19]

Long before Benedict Anderson's *Imagined Communities* (1983), Castoriadis conjured the nation as a particular imaginary formation. For each society, Castoriadis proposes, there is a 'central imaginary' (here we catch echoes of Ricoeur). Its significations represent 'an original investment by society, of the world and itself with meaning', one which orders, values and partly determines 'real' and rational factors.[20] For each society and each historical period, the social imaginary founds or 'institutes' language and the basic institutions of social life. In so doing the social imaginary constitutes for that society 'its singular way of living, seeing and making its own existence', bestowing on each period a quite 'specific ... mood'. And the dynamic process of institution does not stop with the original institution, but ceaselessly continues its work down the generations.

The originary process whereby imaginary patterns of meaning are laid down, Castoriadis calls 'the imaginary institution of society'. In any given case, how might the historian explain the nature of this originary laying down of meaning? While believing the process is finally inexplicable ('ex nihilo'), Castoriadis attaches great importance to conditioning factors which, for a given culture, help shape the role and scope of imaginary significations. Thus to the general influences relevant to, say, a nation, such as language, laws, customs, techniques, arts, topography and climate, for Australia we could add the experience of convictism, the originary power of an authoritarian, centralised state, Anglo-Irish rancour, and race and sex relations. The Australian social imaginary does not operate as a *force upon* these: it *is* these, in the sense that it is the unique patterning or configuration which positions such influences in their relationship to each other and to the whole.

The imaginary institution consists of two moments: the instituting moment and the instituted moment. The instituting moment is the more creative; the instituted moment is the created or conserving moment. In a churning dynamic, the whole instituting cycle repeats and reconfigures itself. Within it, *the instituting moment must always draw on what is already instituted*. This would help explain why, in dilute and complex forms, certain early Anglo qualities have endured over Australia's history. Thus in pursuing the two questions remaining with me after thirty years of writing about identity (the questions of cultural foundation and cultural transmission over the generations), I would now take into account the social imaginary and its instituting process. And I would treat socialisation as a major site of that transmission.

We conclude by considering Castoriadis's 'project of autonomy'. Much of the Castoriadis's last thirty years was dedicated to defining and promoting the project of autonomy which, for him, was what best illustrates the creativity of the social imaginary. Historically, most societies have been not 'autonomous' but 'heteronomous'. Most societies have been 'heteronomous', Castoriadis says, because their members are closed to the fact that the source of their values, norms, orientations and goals lies not with the mythical ancestor, not with God, not with natural law, and not with historical necessity. The source lies with themselves. In ancient Greece between the eigth and fifth centuries BC arose the first germ of such an understanding and hence of autonomy. Infinitely slow, surfacing fitfully and submerging to reappear centuries later, the project of autonomy also involves shared self-government (or moves in its direction) together with the mutual recognition of reflective human subjects (or moves towards this).

If the roots of the project of autonomy are to be found in ancient Greece with the co-birth of philosophy and politics, with the advent of Greek citizenship and its direct-democratic institutions, later expressions of the project can be discovered in medieval burgher challenges to king and feudal lord. Castoriadis saw other expressions of the project of automony in the emancipatory struggles of modernity—in the English, American and French revolutions; in the struggles to establish trade unions; and most recently in the civil rights, women's, youth, gay and lesbian movements.

Standing squarely within the project of autonomy, Australia draws strongly on the creative as well as the conserving aspect of institution, that is to say, on the amazing work of the social imaginary.

11

Psychoanalytic theory and sources of national attachment: the significance of place

Marjorie O'Loughlin

M AJOR VARIANTS WITHIN psychoanalysis have foregrounded the fundamental issue in Freud's work of the relation between self and society.
Psychoanalysis is assumed here to be epistemologically irreducible, encom-
passing a cluster of social theories of great complexity their own right. The
assumption I make in this chapter is that psychoanalytic thought is social in
its very essence and is thus an indispensable tool for understanding the
relationship between the individual and society. My focus here is on the
sources of attachment citizens feel towards the nation and how national
identity is constructed. Acknowledging the importance of fantasy in this, I
look briefly at these issues through what I call an object-relations lens,
notably that furnished by the work of Melanie Klein, Donald Winnicott and
self-psychologist Heinz Kohut. Then drawing upon recent literature which
claims the source of attachment to be either civic or ethnic in character, I
suggest that there is another way of thinking about attachment, one which
is about lived experience grounded in nature, culture and history, but which
avoids sliding into political abstraction or cultural determinacy. Specifically
I explore the imagined relationship between the individual and the nation,
suggesting that ways in which individuals locate themselves in a wider
social entity may be through an attachment to *place*.

The particular concept of place I want to articulate here is not of the
familiar spatial kind, but is rather a phenomenological, embodied place.
As such it is centrally concerned with what Merleau-Ponty called 'living
meaning' and with that meaning-making described by object-relations

theorists such as Kohut and Winnicott. Such meaning-making, I contend, arises out of experiences of embodied receptivity and mutuality that are fundamental to the generation of identity.

Psychoanalysis and social analysis

Psychoanalytic theory probes the 'psychic register' of that 'relentless abstraction' that is the nation.[1] The nation as 'imagined community' has become a powerful influence on recent thinking about social identity.[2] National imaginings or idealisations underlie recent explanations of the ways in which self-conceived nations are said to provide for their citizens the *experience* of belonging. Such accounts also encompass those *symbolic antagonisms* that seem to undermine and limit tolerance and diversity simultaneously as the nation 'holds' its citizens. Rehardening of attitudes towards foreigners in parts of Europe, and reactions to asylum seekers in Australia recently may be seen as examples of these antagonisms at work. Attempts aimed at explaining the processes of attachment to the nation within the individual may therefore shed light on both the positive and negative aspects of national identity.

At its most general, psychoanalysis can be characterised as a particular kind of sensibility, but one which deals with specific forms of feeling, notably those of separation and loss, reparation, omnipotence and fear, resentment, conflict and rivalry. Applied to social analysis it is concerned with those psychic resources which have come to shape social and cultural images and institutions. With its focus on the complexities of object relations in the internal world and exploration of the variety of ways in which internal objects find representation in the external world, psychoanalysis provides a crucial tool for accessing those anxieties and defences which are layered into everyday experience and which are in complex ways foundational to our institutional arrangements—even our law, language and of course our history. As such then, psychoanalytic theory applied to society is fundamentally concerned with meaning creation. As Cornelius Castoriadis reminds us, there is an immensely complex web of meanings permeating, orienting and directing the whole life of the society as well as working through the concrete individuals that corporeally constitute society. A 'magma' of social imaginary significations are conveyed by, and embodied in, the institution of a given society.[3] These social imaginary significations cover the most significant idealisations such as gods, spirits, polis, nation, state and so on. Individuals are what they are by virtue of the social-imaginary significations which make each one so. Crucially, it is the institution of society itself which determines what is 'real' and what is not: whatever appears within or whatever occurs to a particular society has to mean something *for it*. Imaginary significations are such precisely because they are not exhausted by references to the real or the rational but rather come into being through a creative act or process involving fantasy.

The meaning and function of fantasy is without doubt a contentious concept within the various psychoanalytic traditions. Lest it be thought that fantasy's main function is in generating symbolic antagonisms, for example the fear of strangers or hostility to social difference, we need to remind ourselves that in fact it is a major mode of adaptation among human beings. At its most fundamental, it is substitute gratification or compensation for the things we may desire but cannot have—loving families, caring communities, satisfying careers, success in various enterprises and so on. On the one hand fantasies may be relatively uncomplicated expressions of desires; on the other, they may be denials (reaction formations) against conscious impulses. And while they may serve as psychic compensations, they may also serve to heal or erase past deficiencies, injuries and ancient conflicts, or they may act as a hedge against the anxieties and fears produced by a rapidly altering social world. The significance of fantasy for national imaginings is that it creates a milieu of hope for the future, even in the face of apparently intolerable situations. It provides the strength that can enable us to endure. In addition to its crucial function of emotional regulation and self-comfort, fantasy therefore also acts as a rehearsal for future action.

Finally, fantasies by definition run counter to prevailing circumstances and therefore always have a potential for the future. Whatever the motivation that initiates them, they draw on both the memories and the events of peoples' lives and the stories of fictional heroes altering that material according to our underlying longings. But as reworked by the imagination, raw material may be altered beyond recognition—fantasies of the nation for instance, may be beautiful in their perfection but on closer inspection reveal themselves to be made up of fragments often fearful and dangerous. The workings of fantasy are complex and as such deeply affect social life.

Identity and belonging through an object-relations lens

A major understanding since Freud has been that if social and cultural institutions are to endure and to thrive, they must combine authority and restraint with the opportunity for participants to have at least some of their most basic (and primitive) needs met. Another way of putting this is to say that they require adherence to the realty principle while simultaneously compensating us for submitting ourselves to their authority and power. Just as religion, the tribe or clan once exercised this function so now does the nation. The imagery associated with the latter can be grasped as a projective system in which elements of the citizen's inner world are projected onto the experience of nation. In object-relations theory the individual searches for the external embodiment of an idealised object, or we can perhaps see the idealised nation functioning as a 'transitional object' that is operating as a bridge between self and otherness. If we take this further, and instead of idealisations think, with Winnicott and others, of 'good' objects, created by human beings not only as a means of gratification but also of limitation and containment, then the nation is that object which simultaneously represents both satisfaction and reality. It is a kind of 'good object' writ large, saturated with symbol and meaning.

Object-relations theory offers a persuasive account of the interconnections between selfhood, autonomy, gender and social relations. As with the self-psychology of Heinz Kohut it emphasises relational processes as the central indicator of the quality of social life. It is only out of human relatedness that a sense of selfhood can be generated and individual fulfilment realised. But in mapping the relation processes that form the basis for the development/inhibition of the self, such insights can also contribute to our understanding of desired political and social outcomes. In this way certain dimensions of object-relations theory can be used to evaluate the manner in which cultural activities and social institutions may facilitate or prevent authentic communal relations. In object relations, the primary focus is on the interpersonal dimension of desire and its embedding in the structures of social life. Therefore most object-relations theorists to some degree or other highlight the quality of relatedness, the sense of interpersonal bonds and community, and the extent of self-continuity central to evaluating the nature of repression in the modern epoch, the emphasis being away from drive, energies and potential and towards interpersonal issues of social life.

Attachment and its objects

Object-relations theory builds on a well-established set of claims about who and what we come to love and esteem, and what is involved in the rejection of those things perceived as unworthy or dangerous. The attachment to objects is a well-explored theme in the Western philosophical tradition, going back at least as far as Aristotle. Within the European philosophical tradition, for example, the notion of emotional attachment and the suggestion that there might be positive and negative emotions as well as appropriate and inappropriate objects of those emotions is familiar. Further, the idea that our emotional concerns may not find adequate expression has been explored in both philosophical and literary works, and the under-standing that the proper 'play' of emotion is both individually and com-munally grounded has been strongly articulated. The work of both Klein and Winnicott in concretising this show how the objects of what I call emo-tional knowing or feeling-judgements (what Blaise Pascal referred to as the 'reasoning of the heart') are called forth.

Klein posited an originary and unavoidable psychic functioning in which mother and child relate through an unconscious communication of violent, destructive fantasies concerning part-objects and split objects. As the mother is split into good and bad the child's destructive drives are con-tained, allowing for the creative development of projective and introjective processes, regarded by Klein as essential for successful organisation of the self. Where the constitutive hatred is too great, deformations occur result-ing in 'self-pathologies'. But if the process is more successful, good experi-ences are more frequent and gradually the child is led to withdraw those projections of its own destructive urges and to construct the world in more realistic terms. In what is then a depressive position they develop the capa-city to form emotionally durable relationships and to experience others as separate and ambivalent objects. This mode of psychic organisation centres on loss, guilt and reparation. It is integrally connected to that interplay of destruction and reintegration underpinning mature self-organisation. Pain, loss and destruction are therefore unavoidable accompaniments to human relationships.

The broader social and cultural significance of object-relations theory is that it can be applied productively to analyses of such phenomena as attach-ment to the nation, national feeling and identity. Just as the primary care-giver is the perceived source of both pleasure and pain, well-being or its opposite, an analogy can be made with the nation (what Kristeva calls 'Motherlands') as a source of security and nurturance. In the same way that the child with the assistance of the parental superego and the ego ideal creates a good image of itself, so the national image is built successfully or not. If it is unsuccessful, entire societies may find themselves acting out emotions that are based in anxieties about, or even hatreds of, particular segments of the society or groups outside the society which are cast as a threatening Other.

Unconscious transactions involving love and hate, anger and envy, or pain and anxiety occur within the individual but also in the social and political realms. The centrepiece of Kleinian object-relations theory is that it emphasises the primacy of *social relatedness*. This account of human experience—of unconscious intersubjective transactions of love and hate, anger and envy, pain and anxiety—cannot but be relevant to social and political life. Here I follow Anthony Elliot who insists that society should be assessed in terms not only of institutional processes but also with regard to the quality of emotional, interpersonal structures in which people interact.[4] It is in respect of the latter that the notion of the nation as holding its people is developed and applied by Kristeva. She assumes that in our collective fantasies a cycle of reciprocal reproduction involving the nation and human individuals occurs.

Varieties of object-relations theory

Kleinian theory contributes in significant ways to understanding of the self–society relationship. The subject in Klein's account is not only split internally between consciousness and the unconscious, but it is also unavoidably caught up in fantasies of identification with surrounding objects and others. In this account the relation between self and society is particularly fluid and dynamic with aspects of self being both profoundly invested in external objects but also potentially reintegrated into personal life. The notions of projective and introjective identification provide an important means of understanding the complex interpenetrations of fantasy and the real in much of the phenomena that constitutes contemporary culture. This is particularly so in relation to the construction of national identity.

Object-relations theory also shows persuasively that self and Other are inseparably located within one and the same 'package' that makes up the individual. The unconscious other carried around in the 'package' is 'monstrous' and 'persecuting'.[5] It is an Other which matches the fearful, anxious self that constructs and projects it on the world. Much of the imagery of present culture is saturated on the one hand with powerful feelings of paranoia and on the other hand with idealised aspects of the self. Notions of Australian identity in recent years have appeared to reflect this dualism with the nation imagined simultaneously as vulnerable and even fragile, and as robust (masculine?) and self-assured. Perhaps what this reflects is the immensely complicated interplay of fantasy and reality, the processes of destruction and reintegration, fragmentation and reunification that occur in the making of national identity, and the continued movement between love and hate, pain and joy in the mix of positive and negative that is maintained. Thus social meanings and cultural identities are created and integrated only to be destroyed before once more being laid open to renewal.

The social nature of fantasy is revealed in the work of Donald Winnicott and in Heinz Kohut's self-psychology which show how objects from the outside world ('selfobjects' in Kohut) pass into the young individual's own psychic structure furnishing the basis for imaginary experience. Winnicott's idea of 'transitional' space is akin to Kohut's conception of selfobjects facilitating the bridging between inner world and external reality—it suggests a transitional realm from which the infant can take into itself parts of the object in order to secure identity. Through this imaginary immersion in selfobjects the individual experiences the 'feeling states' of the selfobject 'as if they were his own'. For Kohut psychical life contains two kinds of selfobject —that of mirroring selfobjects and idealising selfobjects. Both are important in the construction of identity, but the latter is of particular relevance to an understanding of the power which a sense of nation can exert over the individual. An idealising object confers worth on the emerging self through an investment in the object itself, an object which is experienced as alluring and omnipotent. A fusing takes place with this separate other and it is through the identification with this powerful other that meaning is created. Indeed for Kohut the creation of meaning is essential for both self-creation and for creative and productive involvement with other people.[6]

In Kohut's self-psychology, as in Winnicott's work, imagination transforms psychic reality, enhancing interest, furnishing it with new objects, and inducing it to forge new links between the personal, and the particular and the general. The symbolic construction of a nation therefore involves the ceaseless creative work which our projections do upon the objects of our experience—in the case of the nation the imagined 'good object'. For many citizens there can be a sense in which the most powerful, meaning-conferring object in their lives is the nation. There is all the more reason therefore to try to determine what may lie at the core of this nation; what is the source of the citizen's attachment to it? In the following brief discussion, I identify the two most powerful theories about sources of attachment which draw upon psychoanalytic theories—the civic and ethnic models of the nation.

The nation: civic and ethnic

Conscious of ongoing arguments about the demise of the nation in the face of a globalised world order, Julia Kristeva nonetheless still believes that it is within and through the nation that the economic, political and cultural future of the twenty-first century is to be played out. In *Nations Without Nationalism* object-relations theory is deployed to articulate a theory of the nation as that transitional reality where individuals are held in an identifying space in which they grow and achieve individual autonomy and mature agency. While newcomers are being absorbed, they must meanwhile give way before the general interest which is however expressive of the core culture. In psychoanalytic terms, the civic nation as a transitional reality is for Kristeva the means by which the needs and aspirations of both natives and foreigners can be met. Like transitional objects, such nations constitute an area of play, freedom and creation, offering an identifying and reassuring space for the benefit of all. This is the familiar civic version of the nation. It is also a benign and, in my view, a somewhat rosy view of the civic nation which downplays the extent to which it is basically an abstraction, standing over and above the potential citizen, involving a measure of identification with a political rather than a local, ethnic or some other kind of community to which the sense of attachment may appear more obvious.

It seems to me that Kristeva's reliance on the nation's capacities for holding may place strain on the effectiveness of civic institutions and their ability to consolidate a sense of being held adequately by those institutions. The obvious question is: what happens to the individual and the nation when for a variety of reasons the holding is not adequate? What other source of a sense of belonging is there for the citizen of the modern nation?

This question is answered by the Australian historian Miriam Dixson in a recent work, *The Imaginary Australian: Anglo-Celts and Identity—1788 to the Present*, in which both object relations and other psychoanalytic work is drawn upon to examine how the social structures that constitute the Australian nation hold those individuals living within its boundaries. Dixson believes that 'an ethnic element' has always pre-dated the arrival of the civic nation-state and moreover it has provided 'final, most basic ground' of social cohesion. With the British historian Anthony Smith, she insists that without a prior core of ethnicity with its 'quartet of myths, memories, values and symbols', residing in the main among the ordinary people as distinct from the intellectual classes, there can be no 'transitional object' to hold its citizenry.[7] Thus in her ethnic version of the nation, the Australian nation holding its people through its core culture is associated with a specific ethnicity, that of the Anglo-Celt majority. She maintains that it is within this core culture that Australians will continue to find what most clearly defines them. She supports Smith's argument that any invention of the nation which does not resonate with the pre-existing ethnically based memories, values, myths and symbols is bound to fail, concluding that without a significant prior history of ethnicity there can be neither nations nor nationalism.

Dixson points out, convincingly I think, that the 'habits of the heart' of earlier times live on deeply buried in present generations, shaping present attitudes to ourselves as a community and to political and social issues and problems. She understands history here as the history of *a people* and it is *their* culture, *their* habits which underpin the nation and hold it together. But such a history is replete with symbols and often heavy with nostalgia, ignoring the fact that history actually continues right up to yesterday, and that most people experience it as practical and grassroots living. Moreover people are embodied individuals whose everyday experience occurs *in situ*. Therefore it is only *in place* that the individual is a part of history. The concept of place I have in mind here is a phenomenological one in which place only exists by virtue of embodied selves and is therefore both temporal and spatial, personal and political. In other words it is nothing more or less than the world mediated through subjective embodied experience. Inseparable from this notion of place is that of locality—width, depth, connections, surroundings, 'here, where we are'. It is this sense of place, most comprehensively articulated in the work of the American philosopher Edward Casey, that I maintain provides another way of thinking about the origins of sources of attachment to society and to the nation.

The nation and 'placial' holding

Australia like many countries is made up of localities and regions, rendered such by what Casey refers to as human 'implacement'. Bodies as practico-sensory totalities, through their diverse and complex daily practices, animate and connect all sorts of places, including even the most apparently disparate, ordinary or even unprepossessing places.[8] Lived bodies are the dynamic bond to place—phenomenological, experienced place—where we do things such as earn a living, educate our children, participate in community activities, rest and entertain ourselves or just 'hang out'. As Casey writes, to identify ourselves, to tell who and what we are, we need to fully comprehend where we are, and indeed where we are not. This conception of place is an unfamiliar one because it is really about how space is socialised and how it is always the product of human energy. As such I propose that it provides a possibility for reconfiguring the formation of social and national identity in ways which avoid the focus on a particular people, a core ethnic group or indeed a homeland. It opens up possibilities for 'getting into place' with others and, while treasuring the memories of past 'implacements', always looks to the possibilities future places might afford.

The power of the phenomenological conception of place arise from the very fact of our embodiment. The body is itself a 'protoplace', constituting one's corporeal 'here'. This means that individuals are not simply in a place (a space), rather it is the self, the person, that *constitutes its own place* at any given moment, through its ongoing practice. The key point to note here is that as human beings we engage in such constitution wherever we find ourselves—at home or abroad, amongst strangers, or in the company of family and friends, in so-called empty spaces, or in the midst of the crowd.

Wherever we are engaged in any human activity, alone or with others, we become part of a local 'implaced' population which manifests its own vitality. A particular place possesses us for the duration of the action, whether we are people of the same or different backgrounds, with the same or differing senses of identity, allegiances, propensities and so on. Other people and their practice link me to my place, just as I and my practice links them to theirs. The history of a place becomes *our* history by virtue of our implaced embodied practice, not because it is my property, someone's territory, or our land.

Places are always encultured, no matter their apparent limitations. Such an acculturation is itself a social, indeed a communal, act: we partake of places in common with others, making and remaking them communally. The culture that characterises and shapes a specific place is a shared culture; it is not one that is merely superimposed upon the place, but is rather part of its very facticity. But this does not mean that place is somehow merely natural. If it were, it would not play the constitutive and integrating role it plays in our collective lives. Rather place is already cultural as experienced, and as such it insinuates itself into a collectivity, altering as well as constituting that collectivity. This aspect of cultural plasticity is, I think, what makes place such a meaningful object and therefore a serious alternative to accounts of national attachment which emphasise allegiance to an ethnic or cultural collectivity. Being concerned with enduring, everyday, human implacement the phenomenological version of place offers a vast richness and diversity (as yet largely untapped) of sources of attachment.

Places are very often emotionally contested, as Peter Read points out in his book *Returning to Nothing: The Meaning of Lost Places*. In Australia Indigenous people's mutually sustaining relationship with the land—with place or country—is slowly and painfully being understood by non-indigenous people. But in the phenomenological view of place, all people have powerful attachments not just to land or property, but also to place—rural or urban, extensive or tiny in scope, built or not-built—simply because as human beings, each and every day of their lives they are in some place or other. And all individuals respond individually to locality or place; in other words, they form attachments to their multiple and varied places just as they do with people who themselves are always unavoidably implaced. Thus the sense of belonging is interwoven with attachment, with a sense of being in-place.

I want to argue, therefore, that the analysis of place in the phenomenological sense outlined is particularly important to the exploration of sources of national attachment. A sense of attachment is an important manifestation of the emotional links between individuals and their places. But attachment to place concerns not only positive emotions but also negative ones and these will have deep origins in the early mother–child relationship. The study of place can therefore be illuminated by object-relations theory, specifically by notions such as Winnicott's 'transitional space' and by aspects of Kohut's self-psychology. Embodied place is in essence the endless variety of sites of the innumerable happenings of our daily lives, notably those which allow for relatedness to others and the provision of the groundwork of ongoing imaginative construction. Kohut's account of empathic mirroring and parental idealisations in the making of the infant self-image, and Winnicott's complex notion of the transitional space in which objects of ambiguous status (created and controlled by the infant, or existing in the realm of other people) deal with the relationship between the inner world of fantasy and the outer world of objects and persons. But psychoanalytic theory also reminds us that in lived experience ('placial', embodied experience) the self has no particular duty to accord with logic or rationality, and indeed does not participate in modes of reality that can be described in the vocabularies available in organised social discourse. Rather the phenomenology of the implaced self is to be found in imaginative products, those objects of attachment which, as Winnicott and Kohut would no doubt agree, require imagination to apprehend them.

Object-relations theory and self-psychology can enhance our understanding of phenomenological place as an object of deepest emotional attachment. (Embodied) place, as well as ethnic groups, generates categories, meanings and values that the society needs to conserve. Memory is embodied in individuals and in a broader sense in the social body, but also crucially in place. A historic canon about ethnic origin and culture is not the only thing that is remembered and therefore is not the only thing having the capacity to hold. Corporeal practices which over time form bodily habits and social and ethical dispositions are necessarily, and in a profound sense, implaced. Yet what people have forgotten about those implacements that had nurtured them may not be easily recalled precisely because through our public discourses, our official histories, our institutions and our grand narratives we tend not to recognise this sense of place. But they endure in the imaginary and the citizen's attachment to them are no less meaningful than attachment to ethnic origins. They need therefore in my view to be tapped into and freshly articulated.

Looking beyond both the civic and ethnic models of national attachment to the notion of place seems to me to provide a positive sense of inhabitancy that is central to positive and potentially productive ideas of national belonging. Focusing on the contingencies of our shared life *as lived* and less on our inheritance, however that may be imagined, reminds us of the creativity of human experience and action. In this enterprise those varieties of psychoanaltyic theory I have identified above may prove extremely useful.

12

Contemporary fantasies of ancient hatred: imagining the Yugoslav conflict

Nicola Nixon

To the extent that fantasy shapes representations, actions, and memories, it becomes a crucial component of human behaviour.

Joan Scott, *Gender and the Politics of History.*

WHEN THE COMMENTATORS and observers sought to explain the wars which have dissolved the former Yugoslavia into its contemporary successor states from the summer of 1990 onwards, the vast majority of explanations reiterated the notion that the source of the conflict needed to be understood as the re-emergence of age-old ethnic hatreds in the Balkans. In seeking to assign a simple cause to the ten-year war in the region, nationalist violence was removed from the preceding context of the economic, social and political crises of the 1980s in Yugoslavia, and was portrayed instead in a discourse of historically determined tribalistic violence. In what came to be known as the 'ancient hatreds thesis', the wars which marked the separation of Croatia, Slovenia and Bosnia–Herzegovina from the new Yugoslavia (Serbia and Montenegro) were assigned the trope 'Balkan wars'. Parodying the expression of the ancient hatreds thesis in the US media from 1991 to 1995, James Sadkovich writes that the Balkans have come to signify a place in which 'vicious tribes lived uneasily with one another, romantic rebellion was common, conspiracy normal, civil wars cyclic events, and murdering one's neighbour nothing special'.[1] 'Balkan' re-emerged in the 1990s as a pejorative term which was used to describe an imaginary cartography in which violent conflict was ethnically and historically determined.

The ancient hatreds thesis was actually not a thesis at all. Instead, condensed into the metaphor 'ancient hatreds' were a number of signifiers, in two distinctly oppositional groupings, which operated ideologically. In the first group, 'Balkans' related metonymically to 'Byzantine, 'Ottoman', 'Turk', as well as 'ethnicity' and 'tribalism'. Linked in the second group were such signifiers as 'Great Powers', 'Roman Empire', 'Austro-Hungarian Empire' and, in this case, 'citizenship' and 'civilisation'. In various ways these predominant signifiers provided the coordinates for the ways in which contemporary events were mapped in a story of empires that took the Balkans as its key other. The discourse of ancient hatreds told a story, therefore, not only of a history of the Balkan region over the past 2000 years, but more importantly of the interaction between an ideal of Western civilisation —as something quite distinct and oppositional to Balkan civilisation—and the Balkans. Often quite simply racist, the endless rhetoric of 'ancient Balkan hatreds' produced a hegemonic interpretive frame through which the events of the various conflicts were filtered throughout the decade-long war.

The repetition of the discourse of ancient Balkan animosities, however, does not merely evidence a well-intentioned but fatally prejudiced discourse. Instead the discourse of Balkan tribalism, which narrated the war as part of a lineage of ancient historic conflicts, needs to be understood as a *social fantasy*. The psychoanalytic notion of fantasy provides a means for envisaging the circular operations through which history is conceptualised and produced through contemporary ideological structures. Through psychoanalysis, fantasy may be understood as a fundamentally social phenomenon, operating in unconscious, habitual social practices rather than in cognitive thought. Intersubjective as well as intrasubjective, fantasy operates to provide the social linkage of imagined communities. In this notion of the phantasmic social bond we can see the divergence of psychoanalytic social theories from those based on liberalism. According to the liberalist conception of the social contract, a group is bonded to one another through common aims. For psychoanalysis, however, common aims are not enough to hold a group together; there must be something extra which binds a group libidinally.[2] Operating unconsciously, it is at the level of the libidinal bond between members of a social group that fantasy goes to work. Social fantasies operate ideologically, through 'interpellating or constructing individuals as the willing subjects of the system of exploitation which assigns them their very subjectivity'.[3] As they are ideological, fantasies operate as moral imperatives which structure unconscious desire and effect social processes well beyond the immediate instances of their expression in discourse. As an ideological fantasy, the ancient hatreds thesis may therefore be implicated in the structuration of the social field in and beyond the former Yugoslavia.[4]

To conceptualise the ancient hatreds thesis as an ideological fantasy means reversing the notion of causality that the theory suggests: that the history of the Balkans is one of wars caused by inherent enmities which continually play themselves out through violence. Instead the fantasy of ancient Balkan animosities must be analysed in terms of the ways in which it is a contemporary phenomenon which has operated *performatively* in the events of the wars themselves. While the ancient hatreds thesis is of no use as such for a direct understanding the causal processes which led to the dissolution of Yugoslavia, as a contemporary fantasy structure, it goes to work in the world—a world which includes the symbolic and political landscapes of the former Yugoslavia. In other words, there are a number of ways— political, ideological, and socio-cultural—in which the fantasy of ancient animosities can be understood to have materialised in the events of the wars themselves. It is in this sense that the fantasy may be understood as performative: as that which tends to produce that which it claims merely to name. Conceptualised as an ideological fantasy, the discourse on ancient Balkan hatreds may therefore be analysed according to its own involvement in the perpetration of violence in the former Yugoslavia. And the drive for this narcissistic civilisational ideal may therefore be condemned for the way in which it is not only discriminatory but also performative.

Fantasy operates both on the level of the imaginary 'I' and that of the socio-symbolic order in which identifications are made. Both levels, according to psychoanalysis, operate according to a fundamental misrecognition. At the level of the social, a fundamental misrecognition occurs when subjects perceive themselves as individuated parts of a coherent and unified social whole. The social is therefore misrecognised because, as Ernesto Laclau has argued, since the unification of the social sphere is ultimately impossible the social has, paradoxically, an *absent fullness* at its core.[5] This misrecognised absence produces an anxiety which fantasy attempts to cover over. Since the interrelationship of the subject and the social is the space in which this misrecognition takes place, the significance of an ideological edifice such as 'ancient Balkan hatreds' is, as Slavoj Zizek has argued, 'not the asserted content as such but the way this content is related to the subjective position implied by its own process of enunciation'.[6] In other words, the staging of a certain fantasy of belonging that relies on a misrecognised social whole should be examined according to the subjective position it implies. Fantasy is 'staged', therefore, according to Zizek, for someone or something—a gaze—which would reflect us back to ourselves in the form of our sense of self, often in the form in which we would find ourselves most pleasing. That is, fantasy plays upon our most narcissistic desires. If the gaze is reversed, as Zizek puts it, away from the portrayal of ancient hatreds, to the position of enunciation from which this discourse emerges, we find a fundamentally narcissistic image of Western civilisation emerging at the end of the Cold War. And among those that are to be found identifying with this image, unfortunately, are the international mediators who, staring transfixed at the mirror of the Balkans, found themselves to be eminently civilised.

In the fantasy of Balkan tribalism, the main referent was not only the former Yugoslavia but also the idea of the 'international community'. In this sense, the discourse of ancient hatreds is also a fantasy of civilisational superiority in which the Balkans became a phantasmic space onto which observers of the conflict mapped their own desired self-image as members of a Western civilisation and that which underpins the contemporary 'international community'. This idealised self-image is to be found in the identi- fication of various discourses with a master narrative of civilisation, from narratives of the Roman Empire to the those of Great Powers which are detailed by the numerous instances of the ancient hatreds fantasy. It is indeed no coincidence that the discourse of 'civil society' has gained such symbolic importance in post-communist political discourses as an organis- ing principle and the means by which various political entities stake a claim for recognition as coherent national bodies and/or members of a European civilisation.

This fantasy of ancient Balkan hatreds which dominated media, diplo- matic and academic discourses operated in the discourses of some of the most powerful figures who were involved in the so-called international peace process: those who purported to be enacting 'international' mech- anisms in order to quell the violence in the former Yugoslavia throughout the 1990s. Their continual repetition of the notion of age-old enmity, com- bined with its reiteration through much of the world's most powerful media organisations contributed to what became a hegemonic fantasy structure through which Yugoslavia was viewed. To take just one example, in a White House media briefing in 1997 Press Secretary Michael McCurry evaded a question on the responsibility of the Bosnian Serb leader, Radovan Karadzic, for mass murder in Bosnia by suggesting that the problems there extended well beyond that of any political party. Rather ineloquently, he argued instead that they 'reflect some of the ancient hatreds that have existed in the Balkans generally and that will continue and likely will always be a very difficult situation'.[7]

It was this fantasy structure which was to play a large part in the mech- anisms of 'international peace' in Yugoslavia. The official peace process, instigated as fighting in Croatia spread into Bosnia in 1991, was undertaken by the Office of the United Nations Secretary-General and the then Euro- pean Commission, which each appointed a chairman to the International

Conference on Former Federal Yugoslavia (ICFY) which constructed and attempted to implement various peace plans. Until 1995 the two co-chairs led the ICFY mediation process while the United Nations implemented peacekeeping forces. The longest serving co-chair of the ICFY, and vocal adherent to the ancient hatreds fantasy, was former British Conservative politician, Lord David Owen.

Michel Feher has analysed the ideological content of the rhetoric of the international peace process in the former Yugoslavia. He argues that the discourse of peace in Yugoslavia must be interpreted in the context of what he describes as the 'new doctrine of the international community' in the post-Cold War era. According to Feher, there has been a common interpretive doctrine that has structured the ways in which the wars in Somalia, Rwanda and Yugoslavia have been represented and understood. These three conflicts share the common fate of having occurred at the historical point of the enunciation of a doctrine which has attempted to define a new international community. The self-appointed representatives of this community, predominantly from US and European governments, projected their idealised self-image of civilisational achievement in a discourse that cast all post-Cold War conflicts as fundamentally tribalistic. In other words, the international community's doctrine on post-Cold War conflicts provided its authorised mediators in the Bosnian peace process the ideological terminology through which the Balkans was to be understood as tribal, while the ancient hatreds thesis provided the fantasy support for this claim.

Manifested in Yugoslavia's case as the fantasy of ancient hatreds, the new doctrine removed the possibility of envisioning these conflicts 'in terms of ideological persuasion and political allegiance', in favour of descriptions which emphasised eternal forces of tribalism.[8] Thus, Western authorities, as Feher points out, went out of their way to 'deny any relevant ideological content' in the political mechanisms which were driving the conflicts.[9] Feher's interpretation of the construction of a new international community proliferated by its self-designated representatives from Western governments and authorities during the 1990s is therefore useful for understanding the ideological underpinnings of the peace initiatives which were undertaken in the name of this imagined community. In this sense it is possible to view the various ways in which the discourse on tribal post-Cold War conflicts (perceived to be fuelled by age-old enmity) functioned within the international community's sponsored peace process as self-fulfilling prophecies which acted to exacerbate the continuing conflicts in the former Yugoslavia.

By obscuring the political nature of the violence in the former Yugoslavia, the discourse of the international peace process obscured, most significantly, the mechanisms of the ideological project of 'Greater Serbia' as well, as to a lesser extent, the more short-lived project of 'Greater Croatia'. Engineered by nationalistic governments in Belgrade and Zagreb and carried out by their subcontractors in Bosnia, Croatia and later Kosovo, these two projects enacted violent territorial expansion in the service of the ideal of ethnically pure nation-states. For Croatian and Serbian nationalism the designation of eternal ethnic divisions—age-old hatreds—was part of an ideological project of violent national expansion. The rhetoric of both these expansionist nationalist projects also relied heavily on the narrative of the ancient hatreds which necessitated the division of the Balkans. In the internal Yugoslavian context, the ancient hatreds thesis provided the fantasy support for an ideology which called for the rectification of ancient wrongs through violence—an ideology which was produced, most forcibly, by the propaganda organs of the Milosevic regime. The fantasy of ancient hatreds in the Balkans is not, therefore, purely a product of Western discourse. The synchronicity between the media accounts throughout the 1990s in English-language media and the ideological projects of Greater Serbian and Greater Croatian nationalism suggests a more complex relationship between the two.

Outwardly, the actions of the international mediators were evoked as working towards peace as opposed to the portrayal of a Yugoslavian impetus to war. However, the striking similarities between the rhetoric of ancient hatreds in both nationalist and internationalist discourses on war in the former Yugoslavia highlights that these two fantasy structures have, all along, been mutually supportive. Not only did the international community's representatives obscure the political nature of the projects of nationalism within Yugoslavia but they also reproduced nationalist propaganda for *their own* ideological ends. It is therefore not surprising to find, as Feher has pointed out, that the officials of the international community and their media allies did not hesitate to borrow the arguments of the instigators of the conflicts as their own.

The international mediators mimicked, for example, the rhetoric with which Slobodan Milosevic portrayed the war in Bosnia–Herzegovina to the international media. According to Milosevic's explanations, the war in Bosnia–Herzegovina was to be understood as a 'civil war' in which there were 'no innocent sides'.[10] For Milosevic's purposes, the notion of this war as a civil war provided ideological legitimacy to the farcical suggestion by his regime and its sympathisers that none of the conflict was orchestrated by the regime itself. Meanwhile, the notion of a civil war provided the international mediators with the rhetorical frame through which they could portray their own actions as impartial. In defining the 'sides' of the conflict, Milosevic argued that Bosnia–Herzegovina was 'defined as a republic of three equal, constituent peoples—Muslims, Serbs and Croats'.[11] Translated by the international mediators into their context, this discourse produced the notion that there were three warring factions which would be dealt with impartially by the inherently non-partisan mediation authorities being, as they were, from the international community. The depiction of these three parties, portrayed by both Serbian nationalists and the international mediators as tribal and full of ancient animosities, provided the underlying fantasy support to the claims of both groups that the borders of the former Yugoslavia needed to be changed.

This had a number of significant consequences for any wider understanding of the escalating conflict in Bosnia. The impetus to being perceived as impartial meant the ethical levelling of the actions of the three parties defined by the ICFY. The first of these parties to which the ICFY referred was the Bosnian wing of the Hrvatska Demokratska Zajednica (HDZ, Croatian Democratic Community), the party that won Croatia's first multiparty elections in April 1990. During the Bosnian war the HDZ was led by Franjo Tudjman, the architect of the project of Greater Croatia which attempted to annex parts of Herzegovina to Croatia with the military forces of the Hrvatsko Vijece Odbrane (HVO, Croatian Defence Force), the HDZ-run militia in Bosnia. Led from 1992 to 1994 by Mate Boban, the Bosnian HDZ were committed to a right-wing nationalist ideological framework that included the attempted construction of an ethnically pure Croatian state in Bosnia entitled 'Herzeg-Bosna'.

Secondly there was the radical Bosnian Serb nationalist party, the Srpska Demokratska Stranka (SDS, Serbian Democratic Party), which held power in the self-styled Bosnian Serb state, 'Republika Srpska'. Radovan Karadzic, who also directed the Bosnian Serb Army (BSA), led the SDS. Aligned with Milosevic's Socialist Party of Serbia (SPS), the SDS was committed to a policy of ethnic cleansing that, through terror and the slaughter of civilians, would produce Serb majorities in conquered territory that could then be annexed to Serbia. This adhered to Milosevic's policy of a Greater Serbia, reiterated in the slogan 'All Serbs in one state'.[12] It was the policies of the SDS, carried out by the BSA, which produced the most sustained campaign of violence in the Bosnian war, including the 18-month siege of Sarajevo and the massacre of over 4000 people at Srebrenica. According to the chief prosecutor of the International Criminal Tribunal for the former Yugoslavia (ICTY), Karadzic is

> criminally responsible for the unlawful confinement, murder, rape, sexual assault, torture, beating, robbery and inhumane treatment of civilians; the targeting of political leaders, intellectuals and professionals; the unlawful deportation and transfer of civilians; the unlawful shelling of civilians; the unlawful appropriation and plunder of real and personal property; the destruction of homes and businesses; and the destruction of places of worship.[13]

The ICTY has indicted Karadzic for the charge of genocide, arguing that he, along with others, 'planned, instigated, ordered, committed or otherwise aided and abetted the planning, preparation or execution of the destruction, in whole or in part, of the Bosnian Muslim and Bosnian Croat national, ethnical, racial or religious groups'.[14]

Despite the fact that in March 1994 the Assembly of Citizens of Serbian Nationality and of Serb Ethnic Origin of Bosnia declared to the international community that they would 'defy anyone . . . to claim to represent all the citizens of Serb ethnic origin' in Bosnia, that was precisely how Karadzic's government in Pale was represented by the international community.[15] David Owen, for example, regularly referred to Karadzic as simply the 'leader of the Bosnian Serbs'.[16]

The third party to which the ICFY referred was the government of Bosnia–Herzegovina, elected in the November 1990 elections. The Bosnian president, Alija Izetbegovic, of the Stranka Demokratske Akcije (SDA, Party of Democratic Action), led the government in Sarajevo. Although the SDA was the main Muslim party in Bosnia at the time, and became increasingly nationalist as the war went on, the government itself advocated a multi-ethnic and secular Bosnia. In the discourse of the ICFY, these three parties were reduced to the shorthand designations—Croats, Serbs and Muslims—and in this reduction the political projects of these entities were ethically levelled. The projects of ethnically cleansed Greater Croatia and Greater Serbia were thereby given as much priority in the mediations as the Bosnian government's pleas for international support for the retention of a multi-ethnic state.

The three-party terminology legitimated the ideological position that the population of Bosnia-Herzegovina could simply be divided into three homogenous and mutually exclusive ethnic groups. Furthermore, the ideological frame of the three warring factions claim meant that the leaders of the nationalist factions were taken as the legitimate representatives of the population. Thus Bosnian Serb nationalist leaders were seen to represent a homogenous Bosnian Serb population, as the Bosnian Croat nationalist leaders were seen to represent the similarly homogenous Bosnian Croat population. Within the ideological structures set out by the ICFY, the main exponents of these nationalist discourses were those chosen by the international mediators to participate in the negotiation process. In choosing to negotiate with these politicians rather than denouncing their political projects, the international mediators provided them with a far greater legitimacy than they had previously enjoyed within Bosnian politics. As Feher has argued:

> As soon as they met the demands of the international mediators . . . the so-called faction leaders immediately acquired a legitimate place in the process of

reconstruction ... By virtue of their signature on the peace treaty and their solemn commitment to the establishment of the rule of law, they even became the agents of their country's stability and the guardians of its new institutions.[17]

By mirroring the ethnicised rhetoric of nationalist politicians in Bosnia, the international community reproduced the suggestion of both Serbian and Croatian nationalists that the Bosnian government was an ethnically homogenous 'Bosnian Muslim' entity. David Owen, for example, described the government as 'a Muslim government for a predominantly Muslim population'.[18] As Sabrina Ramet has argued, from the earliest negotiations: 'The U.N. and EC mediators, along with the Western media, began to treat the Bosnian government as if it represented only Muslims, even though, as of 12 February 1993, the Bosnian cabinet still included six Serbs and five Croats, alongside nine Muslims'.[19]

Among the key elements in the fantasy of Serbian nationalism was one that suggested the innate superiority of the 'Serbian civilisation' through a narrative in which the Serbian nation was represented as the last outpost of the defence of European civilisation. Underlying this narrative was an ideology of racial discrimination in which the key signifiers were Kosovan 'terrorists', Croatian 'ustashe', and Muslim 'mujahadeen'. It was against these phantasmic foes that Serbian nationalism portrayed itself as a moral imperative. By the time of the Dayton peace talks, the degree to which the international mediators had integrated the Serbian nationalist perspective into their ideological rhetoric was exemplified by the fact that they 'agreed to partially compensate the Bosnian Serbs for the loss of an ethnically pure Greater Serbia'.[20]

The notion of three Balkan tribes which informed the mediation process from the outset failed to recognise the political and social processes of ethnicisation which were taking place throughout the former Yugoslavia in the 1980s and 1990s following the massive economic crisis in the early 1980s. This process of ethnicisation relied on the redrawing of boundaries, not only symbolically but also materially: reconfiguring communities according to new standards of membership based on ethnicity. Indeed many of the earliest victims of the war were those who could not or would not define their identity along ethnic nationalist lines and many of those who continued to identify themselves as 'Yugoslav'. The violence wrought by these structures has also meant that many people who have opposed the new power structures have been killed, imprisoned, or found themselves exiled from both Croatia and Serbia as national traitors.

The principle of ethnicity also informed the ways in which the international mediators envisaged peace in Bosnia. The guiding idea of the mediation efforts from their earliest manifestation, as David Campbell has suggested, was that 'although Bosnia would be an independent state within its existing borders, it should be partitioned along ethnic lines into three nations'.[21] In this formulation the possibilities for peace in Bosnia were premised on the division of the state into 'three constituent units, based on national principles'.[22] This basic structure was to inform all of the peace treaties drawn up by international mediators and politicians throughout the 1990s. The process through which the international community continually endorsed nationalist political projects that were attempting to violently divide Bosnia and parts of Croatia manifested itself in their policy of cantonisation, based on the ideology of the ethnic homogeneity.

The disingenuous nature of these peace plans is highlighted by the attempt to geographically define the three constituent units. Each plan produced a map of the potential ethnic partition of Bosnia. Ethnic homogeneity and the enforced separation of each of the warring sides were described by negotiators as the only possibility for stability in the region. Bosnia was to be divided therefore into ethnic cantons, to be secured by what was euphemistically termed 'population transfer'. A working group was set up to define these units using Yugoslav census data from 1991. It was these 'constituent units' which were then to become the 'cantons' of subsequent peace proposals. The Vance–Owen peace plan drawn up in January 1993, for example, desired the division of Bosnia–Herzegovina into ten ethnically defined provinces. According to this plan, Bosnia would be divided into nine ethnically constituted units and the capital district of Sarajevo. Each of the warring parties would have a majority in three of the nine provinces. The district surrounding Sarajevo was considered by the international community to be a *de facto* Muslim province. Although the plan was inevitably unsuccessful with the refusal of the Bosnian Serb government to sign, the Vance–Owen plan would have meant the so-called transfer of forty-three per cent of those designated Bosnian Serb, forty-four per cent of those designated Muslim and thirty per cent of those designated Bosnian Croat.[23] Yet the international mediators, in particular Vance and Owen, refused to believe that there could be any other guiding principle besides a geographically designated ethnic homogeneity, based as it was on their belief in a tribalist Balkans.

David Owen, as co-author of the Vance–Owen plan, argued that this would restore a unified, multi-ethnic Bosnia. However, his notion of multi-ethnicity, based as it is on ethnically homogenous cantons, is comparable to a politics of what Etiene Balibar has termed 'meta-racism'. Balibar argues that meta-racism is a form of racism 'whose dominant theme is not biological' but rather 'the insurmountability of cultural differences'.[24] It is 'a racism which at first sight does not postulate the superiority of certain groups or peoples in relation to others but "only" the harmfulness of abolishing frontiers, the incompatibility of lifestyles and traditions'.[25] By postulating that 'individuals are the exclusive heirs and bearers of a single culture' meta-racism serves to lock 'individuals and group . . . into a genealogy, into a determination that is immutable and intangible in origin'.[26]

As Balibar has argued, behind such a situation lies 'barely reworked variants of the idea that the historical cultures of humanity can be divided into two main groups, one assumed to be universalistic and progressive, the other supposed irremediably particularistic and primitive'.[27] With ethnicity as the organising principle, the process of international mediation therefore attempted to institutionalise a form of racism as an anti-racist solution. The international community's insistence on envisaging some kind of eternal ethnic entities as the solution to the Bosnian conflict effectively relegated the complexity of a multi-ethnic Bosnia to the status of an anomaly. And it went further. By euphemistically terming their aim 'population transfer', the various peace plans succeeded in legitimising and exacerbating the politics of ethnic cleansing which they claimed to be preventing. A tragic irony of the Bosnian war is that the violence of ethnic cleansing operations carried out by Serb and Croat nationalist forces in the region was what created the basis for cantonisation of Bosnia along ethnic lines.[28]

So not only did the international mediators legitimise the violent nationalist rhetoric of the politicians of the former Yugoslavia but, according to Kemal Kurspahic, it was often the maps themselves that fuelled campaigns of ethnic cleansing. He argues that when these maps were first introduced into the negotiation process in Lisbon in March 1992, 'Serbian forces started an intensive campaign to "cleanse" the territory designated on the maps as theirs'.[29] They saw their violence as having been legitimised by the international community and 'embarked upon yet another campaign of killing, raping, imprisoning and expelling all non-Serbs'.[30] Similarly, the maps drawn up by the international mediators assisted in destabilising the often-fragile coalition of the HVO and Bosnian government army. Noel Malcolm has suggested that the planned division of Bosnia into ethnic cantons in 1993 'gave local commanders in central Bosnia the idea that they should carve out their own pure ethnic territories, thus turning what had hitherto been only occasional conflicts between Croats and Muslims into a large-scale war'.[31]

While there were many adherents to the ancient hatreds thesis among journalists and politicians, it was the international mediators, therefore, who contributed the most to proliferating ideologies of nationalist expansion in the former Yugoslavia, providing them with both material and discursive shape. Once the ideological ruse of a self-generating tribal conflict is removed from analyses of Yugoslavia's demise, as Zizek argues, it becomes apparent that the international community was from the very beginning involved in the escalation of violence. As Feher proposes, 'while ethnic hatred was not the cause of post-cold war conflicts, it ended up being the main consequence of the policies applied by the international community'.[32] Internal fantasies of nationalism and external ones of civilisation *together* formed a hegemonic ideological structure which legitimised and effected the violent destruction of Yugoslavia. And in the end, it was Serbian nationalism that most effectively staged a spectacle of violent, archaic ethnic passions that fascinated and transfixed so many observers in its narcissistic reflection.

Text and trauma

13

'Impossible history': trauma and testimony among Australian civilians interned by the Japanese in World War II

Christina Twomey

IN 1957, AGED 43, Mrs Grace Kidd[1] described the legacy of her internment by the Japanese during World War II:

> I have the greatest difficulty holding down office jobs of the clerical order or shop jobs because they entail so much figure work, & at times my mind becomes a complete blank. I state that this is directly due to the severe blows on my head which later resulted in blackouts, depression, severe headaches and the inability to handle, at times, the simplest of jobs ... I am in constant fear of losing my job, on which so much depends. My companions at work and my boss have noticed my 'careless' mistakes with quizzical expressions, not knowing that there are times when my mind melts into soft black velvet. I find myself in this engulfing mass, struggling desperately to push it aside and come back to clarity of mind and vision.[2]

The war experiences of internees like Grace Kidd have been virtually forgotten in Australia, where the dramatic and deeply unsettling experiences of military prisoners of war have overshadowed their civilian counterparts. Civilian internees have been largely absent from public commemorations of the experience of captivity in the Pacific War. They have also received scant attention in the historical literature of Australians at war.[3] The Japanese Imperial Forces interned over 1500 Australian civilians, along with thousands of others from Allied nations, in detention centres throughout the Asia-Pacific. Accommodation in the camps ranged from converted university campuses to open-air 'atap' huts.[4] Grace Kidd's statement of her continuing anguish almost a decade after her release from Singapore's Changi internment camp forms part of an extraordinary and unexamined archive of testimony from Australian civilian internees about their war experiences. Mrs Kidd's evocative description of the 'engulfing mass' that threatened to overwhelm her was the plea of a woman traumatised by war. This essay asks if the trauma experienced by Mrs Kidd and others like her can be considered historically specific, and explores how psychoanalytic approaches to trauma might assist in that task.

Trauma and history

'Trauma' itself is a loosely-defined and contested concept, one that challenged Freud and continues to confront psychoanalysis as a pathology unusual in its literality. There does seem to be general agreement among psychiatrists that traumatic symptoms include

> a response, sometimes delayed, to an overwhelming event or events, which takes the form of repeated, intrusive hallucinations, dreams, thoughts or behaviours stemming from the event, along with numbing that may have begun during or after the experience, and possibly also increased arousal to (and avoidance of) stimuli recalling the event.[5]

Broad agreement on the symptoms of trauma has not led to consensus in theorisations of it among psychoanalysts or cultural critics interested in applying psychoanalytic models. Debate has centred on whether the origins of trauma are located within or outside the psyche. Dominick LaCapra is adamant that there is in fact an important distinction to be drawn between structural trauma and historical trauma. Everyone experiences structural trauma—'in terms of the separation from the (m)other . . . the entry to language . . . and so forth'—he insists, but historical trauma is specific and 'not everyone is entitled to the subject-position associated with it'.[6] LaCapra's work has been centrally concerned with the Holocaust, but his insights can be applied usefully to the experiences of civilian internees of the Japanese. They too, in their wartime experiences of detention, neglect and in some cases physical abuse, experienced a set of circumstances that amount to historically specific trauma.

Trauma poses a challenge to psychoanalytic theory precisely because the pathologies that constitute it are *not* distortions of other repressions, wishes and fantasies. The flashbacks, insistent memories and dreams that so disturb the traumatised individual are usually key events or anxieties directly and explicitly related to the traumatic episode. According to Cathy Caruth, the pathology of trauma lies in the reception of the event, which is 'not assimilated or experienced fully at the time, but only belatedly, in its repeated *possession* of the one who experiences it. To be traumatised is precisely to be possessed by an image or an event'.[7] This delay between the traumatic event and its return, which Freud described as 'latency', also means that knowledge of the event has not been fully possessed by the individual. Some civilian internees, for example, did not experience panic attacks or other symptoms of trauma until many years after their liberation. Eve ten Brummelaar, a Dutch woman interned in the Dutch East Indies who later migrated to Australia, recalled: 'Around 1973, I discovered that some outwardly normal situations could plunge me, quite suddenly and without warning, into an acute state of anxiety'.[8] Caruth further suggests that trauma is a 'symptom of history' and that the traumatised 'carry an impossible history within them, or they become themselves the symptom of a history they cannot entirely express'.[9] This tension between the assimilated and unexpressed elements of an individual's past is reflected in Mrs ten Brummelaar's description of feeling like 'two totally different persons. One a cool, calm and collected woman, looking with amazement and disdain at this other creature going to pieces for no apparent reason'.[10]

Considering this notion of an unexpressed history, theorists and psychiatrists working in area of trauma and memory often note the importance of witnessing, or listening by another, to pass out of the sense of isolation imposed by the experience of trauma and begin the process of recovery. Dori Laub, a child survivor of the Holocaust, has written about 'the imperative to tell' and considers that 'no amount of telling ever seems to do justice to this inner compulsion'. For Laub, it is the ' "not telling" of the story that serves as a perpetuation of its tyranny'.[11] Bessel Van der Kolk and Onno Van der Hart state that for a traumatised person to recover, the story must be told in order for the experience to be integrated into the life history, autobiography and personality.[12] It is through witnessing and speaking about and of the past that the impossible history of a trauma is realised. The impossible becomes possible, the history becomes just that, the past, now fully incorporated into the present rather than returning insistently and unbidden to it as an alternative reality.

Historians who find psychoanalysis instructive have tended to adopt its theorisation of ambivalence and distortion as among its most useful tools. In the case of trauma, however, where literal rather than displaced meaning dominates, it is the insistence on witnessing and listening as the pathways to recovery that opens avenues of inquiry for a historian. It is important to ask historical questions about the type of social practices and discourses that enable speech and encourage listening. To put it another way, witnessing can only occur when there is a receptive audience for the tale one has to tell. This insight is particularly useful when it comes to understanding the difficulties former civilian internees faced in the postwar world. The trauma they had experienced was specific, and their fears and anxieties were frequently literal replays of traumatic events endured during their internment. Yet opportunities for discussing and absorbing the meaning of those experiences were limited in a postwar society which discouraged people from dwelling on the past.

A captive audience: the Civilian Internees Trust Fund

In 1952 an opportunity for civilian internees to describe their wartime experiences came from an unlikely source. In that year the Menzies government established the Civilian Internees Trust Fund. The fund oversaw the distribution of money from frozen Japanese assets among Australian civilians or their dependents who had experienced 'distress or hardship' leading to a 'permanent disability', as a result of their internment during the war.[13] In its ten years of operation the trust distributed over £44 000 to eligible applicants.[14] Hundreds of Australians wrote to the trustees, not confining themselves to the official blue foolscap forms that allowed them a few inches of space to describe years of pain. The entreaties and detailed letters that make up this archive, assembled in the 1950s, reveal the continued suffering of some non-combatants long after the war was over. The applications demonstrate the difficulties doctors, the trustees and former internees had in articulating the mental anguish that resulted from internment in the days before psychiatrists gave such symptoms a name: post-traumatic stress disorder. They also show the anomalous place that civilian internees occupied in dominant narratives about war, the nation and sacrifice and for some individuals this compounded their sense of having experienced an impossible history for which it was difficult to find an audience in the 1950s.

The possibility of gaining financial compensation from the trust and the fact that grants were conditional rather than determined on the basis of internment alone might have influenced the terms in which former internees wrote about their experiences of captivity.[15] The wording of the application form encouraged internees who wished to receive a monetary grant to exaggerate the distress or hardship they might have experienced. This financial context means that the internees' testimonies are not unmediated nor are they completely voluntary. Many applicants, however, could not contain themselves within the official forms, nor did they confine themselves to strict descriptions of their disability. 'We very nearly did not come out of that internment camp alive', Mavis McKenna wrote. 'Every night, towards the end, when I kissed my daughter good-night I wondered if she would be alive in the morning. Only those who were interned under similar conditions could understand how long it took to put the war and the Japanese out of our minds'.[16] Letters such as this convey the depth of feeling of some applicants, and their frustration that the suffering of internees received so little recognition in postwar Australia. This suggests much more than mercenary grandstanding. Comparing the lot of civilian internees with their better known military counterparts, Mrs Evelyn Ross stated that 'Civilian Internees . . . lost their homes, personal belongings and still suffer ill-health (no less than the P.O.W.'s)'.[17]

The applications to the fund demonstrate that there is no homogenous traumatic experience, nor does the same event or occurrence traumatise everyone equally. Rita Roberts, a missionary and nurse who had been interned in Lungwha, China, when she was in her mid-forties, worked as a nurse in Tasmania after she returned to Australia. She wrote breezily: 'I have not suffered any "hardship". If, in the future, the secondary anaemia which I have had since internment, prevents me from earning my living I know that my heavenly father will, in some way, meet the need'.[18] Similarly Rose Turnbull, Vice-President of the Australian and New Zealand Association in Singapore before her internment in Changi, concluded after reading the application form that it would be unfair of her to claim money that others may need more than she. Now widowed and living in Melbourne, Mrs Turnbull reported that she was 'not in "dire distress"'.[19]

In contrast, another who had been interned in Shanghai along with her 3-year-old son but separately from her husband, reported constant suffering since war's end. By 1953 she had been hospitalised four times, tormented by 'acute mania'. In 1950 she had twice received electro-shock therapy. All the doctors and psychiatrists reporting on her case pointed to the patient's $3\frac{1}{2}$-year internment as the cause of her mental instability. The woman's husband wrote on her behalf: 'She is avoiding discussion on the life in the camp in general. Dr Mahon expressed an opinion that she might have been bashed or assaulted by Japanese causing extreme mental depression'.[20] Miss Bettina Baker, who had been interned in Changi, told the trustees that she lived in the Melbourne bayside suburb of St Kilda but suffered from 'nerves' and was 'unable to take a position in the city or anywhere where there are crowds'.[21]

Depression, anxiety, and 'nervous' disabilities, tensions and breakdowns were all words that former internees used to describe their continued suffering. 'Trauma' was not a word in common usage in the 1950s, and neither internees nor their medical practitioners used it to describe the legacy of their war experiences. Evelyn Ross, Melbourne-born but a long-term Shanghai resident before her internment, described in layperson's terms the process that Freud identified as the 'latency' inherent in trauma:

> People who had 'physical' disabilities didn't live to tell the tale—and ... the 'disabilities' we suffered were 'mental'—and therefore not visible to the naked eye. People say 'you want to forget internment camp'—how can we, when these so very 'personal' things keep cropping up? ... Who can, therefore, say when and where results of those years of internment will strike us?[22]

Evelyn Ross raged against the restrictive terms of the trust, but other former internees merely noted with sadness the anxieties that plagued their daily lives. Clare Jamison stated that she was a 'nervous wreck' as a result of her internment in Singapore. The postwar years had not been kind to her; in the 1950s both she and her husband were unemployed and living in a tent in Tarragindi, Queensland. 'Starvation and mental torture has left its mark on me for life and made me a broken wreck', she told the fund.[23] Helen Turner, whose husband Paul, a Gallipoli veteran, had died in their Philippines internment camp, described herself as suffering from 'periodical nervous debility and collapse directly due to the hardships and malnutrition suffered in camp'.[24] Amy Macklin claimed to have suffered a 'nervous breakdown' during the war when the Japanese searched her home in Shanghai and stole her possessions. Since war's end she had been 'unable to do any work in particular as I lose my memory often & have to rest in bed for some days. Dr Nordioni said there was no medicine he could prescribe for a cure'.[25]

General practitioners and psychiatrists who wrote to the fund on their patient's behalf often attributed their physical symptoms to unspecified 'nervousness'. Mrs Stella Forgioni was a British subject who had married her now-estranged Australian husband in Shanghai before the war. ('I can assure you that Mr F. . .'s family arrived in Australia before 1843 and we are not "New Australians"', she insisted.) In relation to her internment, she stated:

> I cannot claim that I am incapacitated by loss of any limbs through the Japanese—and I know I only survived because I was healthy and strong when we started our imprisonment. I know too that I have not come out of those bad years of starvation and fear without any marks or trace of the ordeal. When the gates of our camp were opened by the Americans I was flat on my back for six weeks because my heart was behaving very strangely, and it has been the same ever since.[26]

The doctor's certificate that Stella Forgioni included with her application stated that she still suffered from 'palpitations and pains in the chest' and that there was 'a large nervous element in her condition'.

In keeping with the psychoanalytic insistence on the unusual literality of traumatic symptoms, many former civilian internees continued to experience pain and discomfort long after doctors could find any continuing physiological reason for its occurrence. Mrs Delia Hewitt, for example, had suffered from persistent vomiting and insomnia since her internment in Shanghai. By the 1950s her marriage had also broken down, and she was living in Sydney and now over seventy years old. Her long letters to the fund are full of pleadings and a sense of injustice, written in smudged blue ink on fine sheets of pale paper, replete with much jabbing and underlining. She informed the fund that she was 'nervous and unable to sleep & vomit[s] nearly every day'. The doctor who treated her stated that Mrs Hewitt had lost 68 pounds (31 kilograms) while an internee and that 'there has been persistent vomiting & insomnia for a very long time probably of neurologic origin. Nothing could stop her vomiting sometimes. Luminal and morphine injections were sometimes useful to induce her to sleep'.[27] Mrs Ida Spence was another ageing internee who lived at the New South Wales Home for Incurables. The medical officer at the home reported that:

> When an internee she is reported to have suffered much in the way of beatings and kickings by the Japanese, & she constantly complains of pains in her back & right kidney. These pains are not related to her cerebral tumor, & her constant suffering & obsession with them is undoubtedly due to ill-treatment during her internment.[28]

While some former internees experienced the legacy of camp life as repeated behaviours and pains that recalled actual events and illnesses of captivity, for others the trauma appears to have been of a more abstract nature. For them internment represented the transition from privilege to poverty, and this loss was keenly felt. Some of the most 'nervous' women who wrote to the fund were those who had led a once-privileged life in expatriate communities or British colonies, and now found themselves relatively impoverished. These were women widowed when their husbands died during internment or shortly after, or those who remained responsible for the support of young children with the added burden of a permanently sick or incapacitated husband. Mrs Ada Ingerson, for example, was an Australian woman who had married a Dutch planter, then spent the war years interned in a Javanese village. 'Everything we possessed had been taken from us', she told the trustees, 'we had to start life again "from scratch" when the war ended in 1945'. Her husband's health had been ruined by his time as a POW and Indonesian independence also terminated their dreams of returning to the plantation lifestyle. In 1957 they were living on a heavily mortgaged farm in Queensland and Mrs Ingerson had only 'just recently been in hospital because of nervous disorders'.[29]

Grace Kidd is the most eloquent of the correspondents for whom internment represented not just the loss of freedom but the loss of their status and position in life. Mrs Kidd provided the trustees with detailed descriptions of her prewar life in Singapore 'where we had a home and a business of our own'. Health problems and increased competition from 'Asian businessmen' in the postwar period meant that the Kidds failed to re-establish their 'once-flourishing livestock and fodder business'. The family migrated to Brisbane. By the mid-1950s her husband was in his seventies and, according to his wife, an 'old, frail and broken man' who suffered from 'gallstones, ulcers and heavy mental depression' and cancer of the tongue. Their previously privileged life in Singapore was now a distant memory. It is significant that Mrs Kidd's experiences of 'black velvet' and the 'engulfing mass' happened when she performed menial work, her daily reminder of all that she had lost as a result of the war, and her much-reduced circumstances.[30]

Some civilian internees exhibited symptoms of trauma, but others articulated their longing for that which psychoanalytic models suggest is so critical to recovery from trauma: a willing audience to hear them out. Mrs Maree Walker-Lee, whose husband was formerly a health inspector in Shanghai, is one individual who expressed her frustration at the way civilian internees struggled to receive a hearing within government and bureaucratic circles. Her husband had died within five years of their release from internment in China, leaving her a widowed mother, not yet thirty years old, of four children. She complained:

> All my efforts to obtain some small measure of our family rights, which were taken away by the war, has only resulted in one official Department passing the buck on to another Department, and I am getting very tired of it, I do not want anything for myself, but I do want something for the children, even if only sufficient for a deposit on a small home, to give us some measure of security. It is not easy for a woman with 4 young children to entertain ideas of remarrying.[31]

Mrs Walker-Lee's difficulties were not merely bureaucratic. Civilian internees struggled to find an audience because they found themselves in a highly ambiguous position when it came to dominant understandings about participation in war, the nature of sacrifice, and entitlements to compensation for suffering. By the mid-twentieth century in Australia there was a well-developed language that linked military service, sacrifice and the nation. The defence forces were expected to protect the nation and embody its values; their personal suffering was a sacrifice made out of duty to the nation. There was also a less prestigious but nevertheless identifiable tradition of celebrating those who had contributed to the war effort through essential service, economy and charity on the home front. The ground was less certain for internees—civilians who had not been at home, had not played a direct role in battle, but did have direct contact with the military enemy. More significantly, civilian internees had personally suffered hardship, privation and loss at the hands of the Japanese, but were not military personnel in service of their country. Their relationship to discussions about national sacrifice was in the 1950s tenuous at best.

Mrs Walker-Lee was one of the few internees to mention her frustration with the ambiguous position of civilians to the Civilian Internees Trust Fund; might others have felt that the fund was an organisation that would, at last, hear them out? There had been other occasions on which internees had expressed their anger and disappointment at their equivocal position in the eyes of their government. Some internees from the Philippines, among the first released from their camps, had corresponded over this issue in mid-1945. On arrival in Australia, the internees discovered that they had been billed personally for their repatriation to Australia after release from their internment camps. Mrs Mavis McKenna, who was almost forty when she was interned at Santo Tomas in Manila, along with her husband Fred, an AIF Gallipoli veteran, and daughter Joan, was infuriated.[32] The circumstances of the McKennas' homecoming after the war were very different from the holidays home in Australia the family enjoyed in the 1930s, when they were often accompanied by their Filipina amah.[33] In 1945 they arrived in clothing supplied by the Red Cross, and had been malnourished for three years. Newspaper photographs taken of the McKenna family in April 1945 show their bewilderment and displacement. Fred McKenna was photographed at Sydney's Central Station, towering above a sea of elderly women in hats, his gaunt face with its unspeakably sad and haunted eyes staring directly into the camera lens. His daughter Joan appears as a tall, thin girl carrying a blanket tied with string and small hessian bags, belongings crucial in an internment camp but out of place in metropolitan Sydney. The wrists that poke out from her donated cardigan are almost unnaturally tanned and thin.[34]

In the same months these photographs were taken, the McKennas were informed that £250 had been deducted from their account at the Bank of New South Wales for the costs of repatriation. Fred McKenna was outraged, and wrote furious letters to the relevant authorities. He informed the Federal Treasurer that General Blamey had made a personal visit to Santo Tomas internment camp. Blamey had informed the Australians present that their government had arranged for repatriation; no mention was made that the newly liberated internees would be responsible for the costs. Mr McKenna also wondered how the Federal government could turn a blind eye to the sufferings of Australian citizens affected by war. 'It does not seem fair', he wrote in May 1945, 'that Australia which is funding £12,000,000 for a lot of foreigners who have suffered the horrors and ravages of war is treating so meanly its own nationals who have suffered just as horribly'.[35] In the end, and after some negative publicity in the newspapers portraying the government as parsimonious and insufficiently sympathetic, the Commonwealth government decided that the McKennas were right, and agreed to cover the costs of repatriating Australian nationals after their release from the camps.[36]

The Commonwealth government was to hear frequently from Mrs McKenna over the coming decade. By the early 1950s the Prime Minister's Department described her as 'one of our chronic complainants'.[37] Yet far from merely complaining about her situation, Mrs McKenna also detailed the dissolution of her marriage—her husband and daughter now lived in Canada—and her own precarious mental health (she had suffered a 'nervous breakdown'). Mrs McKenna also considered that she and her family had been 'in the front line' during the reoccupation of the Philippines, and stated that General Douglas MacArthur 'regarded us soldiers in the front line and commended us for maintaining faith and refusing to co-operate with the enemy'. 'I cannot see', she wrote during the McKenna's dispute about repatriation costs, 'why civilian prisoners-of-war should not be transported home as are soldier prisoners-of-war ... I would have thought that our Government would be willing to help reinstate us'.[38] Mavis McKenna felt that the common distinction between civilians and the military was an artificial one when it came to internment by the enemy during wartime. From the financial details she supplied to the trust, Mrs McKenna did not especially need the comparatively modest grants they distributed. She did seem to need the opportunity to be heard out, to tell her side of the story, to act as witness to a past that continued to cause her grief and sorrow.

The details that applicants supplied to the Civilian Internees Trust Fund about their former lives, their experiences of internment and the difficulties they faced in postwar Australia as they struggled to find a place after years away read as more than merely factual responses to questions on a bureaucratic form. The overwhelming impression that one receives reading this correspondence is that former internees experienced the process of describing their immediate past as both a painful and cathartic act. The loving and fastidious descriptions of all they had lost—lacquered tea sets, embroidered linen, wedding silver, fur coats, crystal wireless sets, individual items of furniture for a long-vanished private school—seem to conjure up a colonial life at the very moment it was swept away. The litanies of suffering both within the confines of the internment camps and in the immediate postwar years are a measure of the limited opportunities former internees had to act as witness to their own painful, and often traumatic, past. There is a palpable sense that former captives have now themselves discovered that elusive captive audience for which they had been searching. A faceless bureaucrat, or a board of trustees with the power to dispense one-off financial aid did not constitute an end to the suffering or recovery from trauma. But for some, the process of witnessing had begun.

In the 1950s civilian internees often complained of experiences, feelings and symptoms that would later in the century come to be seen as typifying post-traumatic stress disorder. Mrs Kidd's image of her mind melting into 'soft black velvet' is one of the most memorable among many accounts that described repetitive episodes of fear, pain and stress. By drawing on psychoanalytic approaches to trauma, it becomes clear that former civilian internees did not merely suffer from incomplete, or inaccurate, diagnoses of their symptoms. These models suggest that an initial traumatic experience can be compounded, and indeed often relived, if the traumatised individual is unable to bear witness to his or her own past. Postwar Australian society offered stoicism and fortitude as antidotes to the sufferings wrought by war; an encouragement to express grief and trauma were the hallmarks of a later period.[39] The broader public exhortation to reticence in the immediate post-war period is the reason why the archive examined here is so extraordinary. It both offered the chance to view feelings rarely expressed in the 1950s and it established an audience, of sorts, for the war stories of civilian internees. This allowed civilian internees to articulate their own war histories and, in psychoanalytic terms, gave them an opportunity to express and thus begin to incorporate them into the present.

14

Let's stop enjoying the Holocaust and make history instead

Esther Faye

IN SOME RECENT newspaper articles, the Jewish-Australian expatriate writer Lily Brett explains her recent and, I would contend, highly problematic 'love affair' with Germany and Germans in terms of a new-found realisation of what it is that connects Jews to Germans, and vice versa:

> I've learnt about the striking similarities and parallels between generations of Jews who came after the period of the Nazi genocide and the generations of Germans, 70-year-olds down. I can see that, really, *we have the most enormous bond*. We're just knotted together ... I mean, both Jewish children and German children grew up with a wall of silence [emphasis added].[1]

> I've met more people I feel close to, more people I admire, more people I can identify with, in the past 18 months, than I have met in all my 10 years in New York ... I have days when I feel quite *at home* [emphasis added].[2]

While I am deeply troubled by the devotional and sacrificial atmosphere that has marked Brett's public readings in Germany and Austria, what troubles me more is her making *heimisch* (too homely and domesticated) what once, she claims, caused her anxiety and dread. I wonder indeed whether the interests of history are necessarily served by making one *family* of the children of both the persecutors/bystanders/collaborators and the persecuted, or by having the past—the question of 'what happened'—restored to us, Jew and German, alike.[3] It is her *therapeutic* use of history that I would want to question, the value of having 'what happened' tamed and reduced to only one of *heimlich's* shades of meaning.[4] The view of history that I wish to promote here is one that does not disavow what is *unheimlich* in *heimlich*, but continues to recognise the strangeness of the bond that exists because of the Holocaust between Jews and Germans, resisting the push towards the redemptive sameness of our shared pasts.

What I, therefore, propose is that the history of our relation, as 'the second generation', to 'what happened' should not be told without taking into account the heterogeneous element that marks the uncanniness of this bond. And in the light of this imperative, the particular historical question that I want to address—with the help of some Lacanian concepts and the work of another Jewish-Australian writer, Yvonne Fein—is whether it is possible for children of Holocaust survivors (of which Fein is one) to not only recognise this heterogeneous thing in their history but to subtract themselves from its masochistic enjoyment. Thus to begin to make history instead.

Paradoxically, it is this very heterogeneous thing that, according to some theorists, comprises history's truth.[5] Within this view, history—as a 'stage' on which the world is constructed 'in accordance with the laws of the signifier'[6]—is constituted through the necessary exclusion of a real and traumatic object of enjoyment (*jouissance*).[7] Briefly, the real is the structural point of impossibility in any and every symbolic system, the point where the signifiers peter out, exposing the void at its heart; this void is the object as real, as *das Ding*.[8] The point where meaning stops thus confronts the subject with the enigma of the Other's desire, with the real object that the Other lacks, and becomes the site of *jouissance* for the subject, an unbearable and traumatic form of enjoyment beyond the pleasure principle. It is, however, towards this real object, or rather its semblants, that the drive for satisfaction always aims, at the cost sometimes of the subject's very life. *Jouissance*, the impossible satisfaction aimed at by the libidinal drives, you might say, is our enjoying ourselves to death—the antithesis of life *and* of the time of history.

'The passion of hate is as firm a bond as love'[9]

I found my reading of Yvonne Fein's novel *April Fool* an unsettling experience.[10] Why, I wondered, had she chosen to tell a story about the continuing effects of the Holocaust on Australian descendants of its survivors as a crime thriller? Why also had she cast the hard-swearing, hard-drinking, hard-fucking April Taub as its detective heroine, a Jewish-Australian child of survivors obsessively committed to hunting down those Nazis who had at war's end so scandalously gained entry into Australia along with the survivors of their persecution?[11] What unsettled me most about this heroine are the sexual encounters between her and her 'Nazi object'. These play out in unbearably graphic detail what appear to be a sadomasochistic *bond* between Jew and Nazi, between April Taub, the undercover Nazi hunter, and Zachariah Rosenthal (Zac) the son of a Nazi concentration camp officer and a Jewish concentration camp inmate who ensnares April by posing as a Jew. His mission in the plot parallels April's: he is as devoted to the task of rescuing all those Nazis whose presence in Australia is now in danger, as she is to hunting them down and eliminating them. In ways disavowed in Lily Brett's recent declarations of homely love, Yvonne Fein's book thus foregrounds the uncanny bond that still connects Jews to Germans.

The questions I want to consider then are first, how are we to read Yvonne Fein's choice of genre? How, also, are we to judge her heroine's obvious sexual overvaluation[12] of the Nazi object embodied in Zac? Do her repeated acts of masochistic submission to the Nazi object keep her enthralled by and in homage to the masterly command that came from her survivor father and that directed her obsession—'Avenge me'? Or do they actually lead her to a kind of symbolic working-through, to a sublimation of her deathly drive for satisfaction? Does Fein's writing, in other words, perform the act of sacrifice before the Nazi object in order to free its heroine, and through her the author, from the very passion of hate that keeps *both* bound masochistically to a past they never inhabited?

If this is the strategy that is played out, then perhaps we can say that Yvonne Fein, unlike Lily Brett, has found a way of maintaining for herself as much as for her heroine a safe distance from the heterogeneous real of history, from the unimaginable and gaping void in the symbolic order that the registration of her parents' experiences of the Holocaust must have opened up for her. If so, then Fein's novel offers us a glimpse of the limited form of freedom that, according to Jacques Lacan, is available to a human subject. This is the freedom, as Freud says, to 'decide one way or the other'.[13] We can either continue to repeat the enjoyment that binds us to a dead past, or we can enter the time of our own desire via the sublimating signifier and begin to make history instead. How we read Yvonne Fein's novel therefore helps us to work through the problem with which I began—the troublesome and deeply ambivalent bond between Jew and German. Is also throws light more generally on the post-Holocaust generation's relation—one of enjoyment or desire—to the historical events that engulfed our parents and which continue to press their claims upon us.

'How can you ever stop being angry at what happened?'[14]

The continuing effect of the Holocaust on this generation has been of interest to those working within the psychotherapeutic field, as well as elsewhere.[15] One of the ways this historical trauma is seen to reappear in the second generation is via their unconscious identification, which could be with the survivor parent(s) as victim, or with the dead that they had lost and/or with their persecutors. Moreover, identification with one does not preclude identification with the other. Even today, the problem of unconscious identification with the aggressor, as one version of the uncanny bond between Jew and Nazi, continues to demand recognition.[16]

Yvonne Fein tells me during our interview: 'I think I was born knowing my father's pain'.[17] She also tells an audience of children of survivors: 'I had to do something about my parents' pain . . . because it was so huge and so painful'.[18] As an analyst asks, 'What do you do with the suffering from a wrong that has already occurred and that cannot be made right? Should one accept such suffering or revenge it, attempt to mourn it or forget it, *do* nothing, but write about it, symbolise it?'[19] For Fein this question resolved itself early in her life as the need to create a mental map so that finally she would know where she was going in the midst of all the pain she had inherited and the anger it fuelled.[20] It also fed her desire to write.[21] At the age of twelve, she began recording in her diary the names of family members her parents had lost in the Holocaust. She knows that she will never be able to redeem the losses her parents suffered, nor assuage their pain, nor exact enough payment from 'the killers of my mother's and father's little brothers' (as April Taub puts it),[22] but she can write. As Yvonne Fein tells me, 'Writing is a way of making it into stories', a way of making 'beauty out of horror'.[23]

Yvonne Fein is not April Taub, but there is more than a 'coincidental'[24] relationship between the fiction we are presented with in the pages of this book and the author who is its storyteller.[25] There is also a personal history and significance to her writing this novel as crime fiction, a genre which she has 'devoured' for the last thirty years[26] and which succeeded her childhood fascination with stories about the knights of the Arthurian romance. Having proposed that it is legitimate for us to claim a historical relationship between this novel and Yvonne Fein, the question that will exercise me shortly is whether this detective novel, which enacts, as I will show, the doomed quest of its knight/detective, succeeds in transforming the horror that feeds Fein's hatred and anger. Does it, in more Lacanian terms, moor the affects of anger and hatred to signifiers that recipher the unimaginable horror? Does it metaphorise the impassable void in her history? Does it in other words help her maintain sufficient symbolic distance from the real thing excluded from it?[27]

For love of the father

A particular set of words and phrases that recur at critical moments in the novel appear to function as determinants of April Taub's quest to pursue those Nazis hiding in Australia. These she remembers her father having written her in a letter: 'You are the last one who cares enough'.[28] 'If you die . . . then there is no-one'.[29] 'If you fail, there is no-one left to exact vengeance. If you succeed, the blood you spill is the life, the death and the burial they were denied. You are the last. You are the last'.[30] We could say that April Taub was driven to join the Nazi hunting organisation K. N. Ripstone Inc.— 'daughter of the persecuted . . . become[s] the hunter of the persecutors'[31] —in response to a command that had come from her father.[32] We could also say then that her life choice functions as *Wiedergutmachung*[33] (making good again), her vain attempt to restore the light (life) that left her father's eyes whenever he remembered 'what had happened'.[34]

The desire implicated here is crudely interpreted for us by April's employer and lover Jake: 'I'm not your fucking father and in the absence of being able to fuck him, you do this for him instead'.[35] It joins her, via a process of identification, to her father's past and to what he had loved and lost:

> Left alone on Saturday nights, too old for babysitting, too young to date, my deepest, guiltiest pleasure lay in examining the contents of the three shoe-boxes I had discovered on a low shelf at the back of the wardrobe which housed my father's not inconsiderable collection of hand-tailored suits. I would snuggle deep into the smell of him . . . and begin. Sepia photographs of children with deep, haunting eyes . . . their ghostly laughter echoing down through the decades to shiver in my eyes . . . I had identified my father in one of them . . . Behind him stood a girl whose face made me tremble whenever I gathered sufficient courage to look at her for any length of time. Without asking . . . I knew her to be the favourite first cousin whom he very occasionally mentioned as being the one he had loved . . . best of all . . . Looking at her face in the photograph was looking at my own in the mirror.[36]

A recurring Holocaust nightmare that always ends the same way for April—with her 'silent scream'[37]—is, however, one outcome of this impossible love. It is a nightmare in which the dreamer finds herself immobilised with guilt. At first her mother saves her—'She won't let me get on the train with her. She gives me to a priest instead'[38]—but in the dreamer's determination to return to her mother the dream ends with the dreamer facing an impossible (and Oedipal) choice. Hence the 'silent scream': 'I will die if I call out; she will die if I don't'.[39] Just as April Taub will dream 'dreams in which Dan [her brother] and I were children again, playing games no children should ever have to invent and swearing an oath that at least one of us would avenge the pain of our parents',[40] so too does her creator, Yvonne Fein, talk of a command to 'avenge' 'this flesh of my flesh', 'to kill the Germans who had killed [my family]', a vengeance aimed at 'lessening the pain of their deaths', at 'assuaging the pain that there is no healing for in the hearts of my parents'.[41] In the context of the 'traumatic screen' of their shared parental 'Mythos of [heroic] Survival',[42] April articulates the author's painful knowledge that her quest to 'right [write] wrongs'[43] is an impossible one:

> To assuage my guilt at being alive and well here, I could spill German blood with Australian-made bullets until I turned the Yarra River vermilion and still the question would remain: how could anything I attempted even approximate the terror and passion, the beauty and obscenity endured by those who had survived?[44]

I will discuss later the significance I attach to the impossibility of her quest to change the course of history, the structural fact that her acts of hunting/writing could never be adequate to their aim. Here I want to explore how her impotence in the face of this impossibility of catching the object of her quest is enacted at the level of what her character April is allowed to consciously know. Something always seems to prevent her from knowing when she is in the presence of her enemy; moreover, its presence induces in her an almost swoon-like state. For example at the very moment when she is, although she doesn't realise this, close to the Nazi she has been obsessively hunting for years, we see her reflecting abstractly on the fact that 'although I was close enough to Wermut to spit in his eye, I had lost the certainty I had been born with as to the true nature of the enemy'.[45] And from her first libidinally charged encounter with Zac, who is in fact this Wermut's nephew, she is placed in the impotent position of both (unconsciously) knowing and not knowing this essential fact; she will only consciously know it later. Fein's plot thus constantly exposes the way that although April does know at some level—the level of her unconscious knowledge—she becomes inexplicably confused and loses the ability to differentiate clearly between enemy and friend, between herself as avenger and as victim. What she, in other words, does not and cannot know until the end of her quest is precisely how close she has been to the Nazi object. Although, as she notes, he infects her unconscious nightly—'I saw this man every night in recurring nightmares'[46]—she does not yet know in what ways the passion of hate that binds her to the Nazi is tied to the fascinating hold her father's commanding script has of her.

We can use April's relationship with Zac to tease out the precise dimensions of her passion for ignorance and the role this theme plays in Fein's own working-through of the uncanny and ambivalent relationship between second generation Jews and Germans. Not unexpectedly, but precisely to the point, April's *body* is shown to hold the key. April has constructed a career and a character grounded in disbelief and defiance of authority figures, which on one level she knows conflicts with her need to please them ('I was always a sucker for approval, especially from authority figures I despised').[47] But what she does not know is why she experiences an uncontrollable 'enjoyment' in her body in relation to the very man whom she already has been given enough reason to mistrust—Zac. Even when, for instance, she is conscious of the fact that he has deliberately manipulated 'some sort of intensity' from her, she finds herself in the position that her whole character and life appears to have been constructed around repudiating:

> We both know it, and even knowing it, I submit. As my body relaxes inside the circle of his arms, my mind goes on the alert: taut, afraid, excited . . . However much I might despise it, submission is the story of my life: submitting articles to Jake, action plans to KNR—all for approval that never seems to come from inside myself.[48]

Where does such submission take her? Inevitably to the very core of what binds her to her enemy and her enemy to her: to the sadomasochistic beating/punishment fantasy that gets played out between them. The narrative shows it beginning quietly at first, with Zac letting her and us know how very much he understands her/his fantasy: 'I'd take you home and undress you slowly. Then I'd touch you very softly on every extremity. You'd have to lie perfectly still while I did it, and not make a sound. If you moved or moaned I would beat you'.[49] Soon enough, however, we see April again submitting her body against her conscious desire, this time to another man who forces on her a punishing regime of diet and exercise. Significantly, the outcome of this is a body that resembles the idealised (fascist) body—lean and spare, muscular and powerful, a phallic tool in the hands of a master[50] —so completely transforming it that she is (as it was intended) not only unrecognisable to her enemy but also to herself. In this instance, her physical act of submission to the master of her training regime is a foretaste of what she will experience again later with that Nazi's son, Zac, as they head towards their final destination, the place in the centre of Australia where the fugitive Nazis are holed up. To him she will submit passively. Submitting without a sound, but not without enjoyment, to the sadistic (sexual) desire of another, bound to him as he is to her in 'that tract of brain and body space that we shared, that wasteland of mutual paranoia'.[51]

So what is Fein's point? Why make us witness these scenes of enjoyment? Psychoanalysis may help us here. As Freud came to recognise, a kind of erotogenic and masochistic enjoyment is *the* primary form of satisfaction that we all aim for, a form of satisfaction that finds its fundamental expression in the fantasy of being beaten, or rather in the need to be punished or humiliated.[52] Or as Lacan formulated it, paying homage to a particular master signifier, that unary trait of identification which is fundamentally 'a mark on the skin', the primary mark that identifies and commands how we are to enjoy,[53] requires that the subject turn herself/himself into an object to be enjoyed by another. Although Freud did not use the terms that his daughter Anna Freud later did, we could say that what this amounts to is that 'identification with the aggressor' is structurally constitutive of the human subject. We could then go on to say, taking the particularities of the subject's history into account, that April's submission to a master who incarnates this primary identification is her way of continuing to enjoy the mark that keeps her bound to the Holocaust. Masochism, the act of engaging the other to beat one, either in fantasy or in reality, is the neurotic's way of ensuring the Other's love; of guaranteeing that the Other exists as absolute, as not divided by the tragedies of history, as not having had done to them what was done to them during the Holocaust.[54]

If we accept this theoretical turn, the question then becomes whether it is possible for any human being, let alone the children of survivors that April Taub represents, to detach herself/himself from the enjoyment that derives from this form of masochistic submission.[55] In relation to the second generation, we might phrase the question like this: what would it take to subtract ourselves from masochistic submission to the master signifier that identifies us? What would it take as well to unfix us from determinedly seeking the real and uncanny object that this signifier points us to? What would it take, therefore, to detach us from our enjoyment of the Holocaust? In relation to these questions, what remains to be resolved is where we are being taken in Yvonne Fein's story about April Taub. It is not only a question of seeing how much April's being '*profoundly* dedicated—to [Wermut's] capture and execution', to 'the cause' is so clearly linked to her hate, to her having simply made 'a career out of [her] pain'.[56] It also concerns more profoundly the question of whether Fein's dedicated quest to 'carry the torch of my people in the unlikely Antipodes'[57] keeps her trapped in a *jouissance* of her hate and anger.

Or has Fein, through the writing of this story, been able to channel the 'murderous impulses'[58] she ascribes to April but which she, like April and other children of Holocaust survivors, is in danger of satisfying/enjoying to death? To answer these questions I need to return to the question of this novel's genre and to ask what kind of act her writing performs.

What drew me to a closer examination of this novel was precisely the question that Fein's choice of detective genre raises about her own relation to the enjoyment of 'what happened'. It is with this issue that I will conclude my discussion. There are several questions I want to consider here. Does her writing enact a masochistic repetition that keeps its author bound to a 'stultifying' beating fantasy?[59] Or does it somehow work through the murderous impulses behind the fantasy to dissolve her fascination with the Holocaust? In other words, is her writing therefore a truly creative[60] and transformative act that allows her to move beyond the fantasy, 'to go on'[61] and begin to make history instead? Let me immediately declare that Fein's attraction to this genre of fiction rests, I believe, on its ability to model the impossible and impotent position that her birth as a child of Holocaust survivors placed her in. Hunting Nazis, uncovering their secret presence in Australia and making them pay for their unspeakable crimes, which the book's detective genre plays out, becomes the vehicle then for the staging of a fantasy in relation to that impossibility. Essentially I think that what draws Fein to this genre are the possibilities offered by its rules and conventions for treating her impotent position, chief amongst which is, as she has said on a number of occasions, that its loner hero is protected from death 'by an unshakeable moral centre'.

> That is the antithesis of what I grew up knowing. I grew up knowing that people with moral centres, who acted nobly died for it and there was nothing that could save them, not God, not their families, not the people who were dearest to them. I found in fiction, characters whose moral centres held and who survived. This became for me the quintessential hero.[62]

Modelling her character April Taub on such a hero is thus Fein's way, she tells me, of satisfying 'a profound and disturbing need to right [write] wrongs'. She refers to this need as her 'John Wayne complex': 'the lone righter of wrongs . . . who found the truth, damn the consequences' and 'yet survived the truth'.[63] In fact, the truth that the hero is really protected from is the truth concerning her/his deathly passion of hate, which, as Freud explained, is older than love.[64] This passion does not so much represent the death drive as point to its place in the subject, the place where the subject enjoys.[65]

Yet there is another feature of the detective genre that mobilises Fein's writing desire. She tells me that she, like April, is a 'lover of doomed quests'.[66] In *The Ethics of Psychoanalysis* Lacan illustrates the psychoanalytic concept of sublimation, in its function as ethic, with a form of literature that is emblematic of such love: courtly love poetry.[67] There are I believe certain correspondences between Lacan's exemplary instance of sublimation and Fein's choice of genre, chief amongst which, for our purposes, is that both concern an impossible object of satisfaction and both enact a set of techniques that defer and ultimately deprive the lover of that real object that would satisfy the lover/detective to death. This work of sublimation, the act of placing a diacritical signifier in place of the non-diacritical mark on the skin, one that 'remembers' where the real object was, thus always concerns something real that must be lost to the subject *if* it is to enter the time of history, the time of the metonymy of desire.[68] The essential point to note here is that in its substitution of 'form for flesh',[69] the creative act of sublimation enables a necessary distance to be kept between the subject and the real of the object, in other words between the subject and her or his enjoyment/ *jouissance*.[70]

I believe this is what Yvonne Fein must be aiming for in her choice of genre. Unlike Brett, Fein's writing seriously attempts to unlock the fascination with the master (the basis of fascism[71]) and the accompanying *jouissance* that keeps many of the second generation bound to the past. Even though the end of the novel has April partially satisfy her death drive in the execution of Wermut and Zac, as she lines up the rest of the geriatric Nazis, the object changes before her eyes and she registers the absurdity of the situation. 'This was what I had dreamed about? Was I about to live out a lifetime of revenge fantasies on these decrepit, pathetic specimens?'[72] The object before her eyes has turned into a decrepit simulacrum of the real Thing (*das Ding*). No longer able to function as a point of identification for her *it* remains unimaginable and inaccessible.

However, it takes one more piece of knowledge for her to register the doomed nature of her quest, and this concerns Jake, one of the representatives of the cause to which she has been dedicated. Jake finally reveals the truth to her: 'I am KNR [the undercover Nazi hunting organisation which recruited April Taub]. I invented it; . . . You're all my people. I love y'all; I need y'all. We fight the fight, kid. Remember Masada? Never again! Never again!'[73] In the shocking recognition of Jake's deception ('I no longer understood the difference between the treatment I had received at the hands of my own people and the rape Zac had consummated upon my protesting unprotesting body')[74] April is finally led to recognise the posturing signifier for what it is—just a signifier. Jews, like Jake, posturing as musketeers; Jews, like her, posturing as John Wayne.[75] That her unconscious knows this before she does is evident in the parapraxis—she calls the Jew Jake by the Nazi Zac's name—which releases her finally from the 'pure culture of the death drive'.[76]

Where to then? How to treat the real that won't go away? I believe that this novel shows us one way out of the static real of enjoyment and a way into history. Interestingly Fein searches for other ways apart from in her writing to enter the time of history: she participates in the ancient

Jewish ritual of purification, the *mikveh*; she reads the Torah.[77] She sees these highly ritual acts as having the power to connect her to Jewish history, but symbolically rather than in the real. There is always the possibility that Fein's desire in regard to these acts is one of nostalgia, a desire for a lost imaginary plenitude.[78] On the other hand, we could read her desire (and this is my temptation at this stage) as her faith in symbolisation *per se*, not in terms of what it can restore but in terms of what it avowedly can't. The only hope I see of freeing ourselves from the masochistic enjoyment of a perfect master signifier, which many of us interpret as a command to undo the tragedy of our parents' history, is by entering the imperfect stage of history itself. In acknowledging itself to be a staged scene with which we treat the real, history maintains the necessary gap between itself and the real thing and allows us perhaps the only kind of subtraction from the enjoyment that keeps us bound together—Jew and German—that may be possible.

15

Narratives, terminable and interminable: literature, psychoanalysis and Margaret Atwood's *Alias Grace*

Rose Lucas

This is not a story to pass on ...

Toni Morrison, Beloved

THE DISCOURSES of literature and psychoanalysis are both centrally concerned with the construction of narrative. Both weave, into recognisable and articulable patterns, the disparate threads of what is externally perceivable, what is absent or silent, and what is available to interpretation by the self and by others. The role of the imagination, or the interpreter, in providing narrative coherence may vary across discourses and textual plots, and there are of course inevitable differences of emphases between texts of fiction and those of personal memory. I would define fiction as the consciously inventive processes of the story-telling impulse which invariably interweaves that which is externally verifiable with that which is intentionally produced. Memory, such as is activated via the processes of therapeutic analysis, is a process of episodic and imagistic narrative-making which is less conscious of the role of the imagination or the unconscious in its own production. In formulating these patterns of narrative—be they linear, resolvable or otherwise—literature and psychoanalysis share a common aspiration: to use imagination or interpretation to offer structures in which to house, and thus to better comprehend and manage, the shifting palimpsest of individual identity within broader cultural and historical contexts.

In the optimistic scenario which implicitly impels the production of narrative, within both literary and psychoanalytic frameworks the telling of stories is the pathway to comprehension and redemption from the oppressive power of what is hidden or repressed. The liberating narrative is the one that would ideally bring about a 'cure' or release from the shackles of neurosis or from the solipsism of incoherence. All, or at least all that is vital, is revealed by the externalising impulses of such a structure: the Gordian knot of confusion, mystery and loss is cut, and the shroud of stasis is reversed, revealing itself as chrysalis, birth site of a new self. In this sense narrative becomes exodus, as we speak and shape our way to freedom from the yoke of the past, and The Story catapults the re-formed subject into the sphere of new potential. As Freud wrote in 1914, the 'aim' of the various practices of psychoanalysis, from its origins in hypnosis to its contemporary praxis in his own time, was 'to recover the lost memories . . . to conquer the resistances caused by repression'.[1] In particular, psychoanalysis as narrative strives to suture the wounds of forgetting, where ' "forgetting" consists mostly of a falling away of the links between various ideas, a failure to draw conclusion, an isolating of certain memories'.[2]

This representation of psychoanalysis is itself an almost mythic story of enablement, albeit one which is perhaps necessary to facilitate the drive or desire which levers the subject, and especially the neurotic subject, out of darkness and inertia and into what is at least the potential for light and wholeness. The iconic goals of 'cure', 'remembering', 'release' and 'integration' may assist in hauling the subject towards an engagement with life and its vicissitudes. The gradual assumption of the active position of speaker, or narrative maker, which is arguably the goal of both the transference process and the production of literature, is indeed a highly significant achievement in any individual's necessarily tentative movement toward subject formation. However, as Freud noted both in *Beyond the Pleasure Principle* in 1920[3] and in his late essay 'Analysis Terminable and Interminable' in 1937, the goals of release and subjectivity through the role of story-telling or the talking cure, while being an essential thread, cannot constitute the 'whole story'. On the *intra*subjective level, the conflicting impulses inherently at work within the unconscious mind will inevitably ensure that the story is destined to remain partial and puckered by absences. For Freud, this fundamental conflict, recognised within the therapeutic arena as a 'force at work which is defending itself by all possible means against recovery and is clinging tenaciously to illness and suffering', could be described in terms of 'the concurrent or opposing action of the two primal instincts—Eros and the death instinct'.[4] In addition, on the level of *inter*subjectivity, as will become clear in the discussion of *Alias Grace*, the mythic goal of completion will be complicated by the story which is always evolving between the teller and the interpreter/reader of the tale. This node of exchange, so pivotal in the processes of reading texts and of transference/counter-transference, will both facilitate and compound whatever narrative is produced.

Such a tension, Freud concluded as his own mortality closed in, condemns the human subject, Sisyphus-like, to interminable oscillations between dichotomous and fantastical positions of wholeness and fragmentation, remembering and forgetting, speech and silence. The narratives of psychoanalysis, therefore, both theoretical and therapeutic, hold out the apparent promise of release and integration, of a full articulation of any individual or individual's story. Yet at the same time they are inevitably undercut by their own primary premise—that is, by the very imbricated nature of forgetting, silence and repression in the 'motley variety' of threads which formulate human subjectivity and the unconscious mind in particular.[5] As a discourse of apparent comprehension and healing, psychoanalysis is thus locked in fundamental struggle with what might be described as its seminal limitation—that the analysis of 'cure' must always be interminable, continually unravelling and being rewoven because, by virtue of the intractability of the unconscious, it can never entirely remove the cancers of resistance and gap.

As a consequence, forgetting or neurosis may not be an alterity invading the pristine integrity of the self; rather the notion of subjectivity itself is necessarily reconceptualised as fundamentally constituted by divergent and contradictory impulses or desires. Instead of requiring the expulsion of the hidden, the goal of narrative itself might then be redefined as the externalised acknowledgement of subjectivity's inevitably complex components of accessibility and inaccessibility. Thus, as Freud himself came to recognise, the talking cure may not be a path to liberation from neurosis, although at its significant best it may offer greater knowledge of the field of the subject, its geographies of surface and depth, its interplay of light and shadows. In this sense, every speech, every narrative formation, is as necessarily filled with feint and absence as it is with revelation and coherence.

This radical rupturing of a model of distinct surface and depth, of presence and absence, is equally apparent within theories about and contemporary praxes of literature. Within a general *zeitgeist* of postmodernity—but also crucially informed by theoretical psychoanalysis's observations regarding the permeable membrane between conscious and unconscious thought—the literary arena is one in which different voices and threads can dip and weave, and in which the putative goal of a conclusion tends to catapult a reader back into the exigencies of plot or text rather than providing any narrative seal.[6] Within a literary narrative that borrows from or builds upon the deconstructive premises in which, as Derrida described it, meaning is endlessly deferred, in which the 'trace' remains an elusive mirage, resolution may not necessarily be reached.[7] 'Clues' may or may not be redolent of externalised meaning, speech may not lead to revelation and release. A narrative *is* shaped, and it provides points of coherence, perhaps even epiphany, but it is also an effort toward meaningfulness which is continually threatening to dissolve, its attempts at integration always under erasure as they are problematised by the emergence of conflicting 'evidences' and voices.

Margaret Atwood's 1996 novel *Alias Grace* is a useful text across which to consider the role of narrative within both literature and psychoanalysis as both discourses are integrally linked within the production of her text. Based around a notorious Canadian case of 1843 in which a young gentleman and his housekeeper/lover are brutally murdered, the novel, like much public opinion at the time, focuses in upon the character of Grace Marks, the young maid who may or may not have been involved in the slayings. As Atwood presents her, Grace embodies a conundrum; beautiful, intelligent, and apparently proper, she claims significant gaps in her memory on the day of the murders. At least according to the surface narrative, even Grace herself doesn't know if she is innocent or guilty, despite being implicated by her fellow servant and found guilty by the law. Atwood uses this lurid puzzle as a device to inquire into the workings of a mind, to conduct with the acuity of an analyst and the licence of a novelist an exploration of necessarily complex human motivation. As readers we are drawn into the web of this curiosity, this desire to pin down and know, and thus by implication, to tell and to hear a narrative of conclusiveness and truth. However, as Freud had noted about the processes of psychoanalysis, the narrative/s which we do find are riddled with clues and doubts, with discoveries and inconsistencies, with the need to repeat and retrack, to speak and to fall silent. Most significantly, it is our own almost unbridled desires as readers to hold fast the truth of identity and individual psychology which are exposed as the narrative sews its myriad quilts of disclosure and erasure.

Consistent with the notion of pastiche and the broadening of the notion of text, *Alias Grace* crosses and destabilises the conventional genre categories of fiction, history, murder mystery and crime detection, and psychological analysis. This is formally achieved by juxtaposing different forms of text—the pictorial, the newspaper report, popular songs, poetry, letters—as well as moving between first person and third person narration. With its bricolage[8] of voices, and yet with a central focus resting both on the exploration of a particular subjectivity—that of the 'celebrated murderess'[9]—and the inevitable, inextricable presence which interprets that subjectivity, *Alias Grace* resembles, if not an analysis proper, then the recounting of an analysis. Indeed psychoanalysis plays both a structural and a thematic role in the production of Atwood's narrative. Most obviously, much of the text consists of, or is triggered by, Grace's psychological examination by Simon Jordan, an aspiring doctor within the perplexing field of mental health. The year he begins his sessions with Grace is 1859, sixteen years after the notorious murders of Mr Kinnear and Nancy Montgomery, and forty-two years before the landmark publication of Freud's *Interpretation of Dreams*. Nevertheless, informed in part by the hypnotic techniques of Mesmer and by a growing European interest in neuroscience, particularly in hysterics, Atwood places Simon at an immediately pre-psychoanalysis point within medical paradigms. While he readily admits that 'the mind and its workings . . . [are still] a *terra incognita*',[10] a geography largely uncolonised by rationality, Simon's techniques of suggestion and association resemble later psychoanalytic technique as first formalised by Freud. Basing his 'scientific' examination of Grace around a series of interviews, he encourages her to talk freely and as broadly as possible, while also seeking to guide her revelations by the use of various prompts—an apple, root vegetables, a candlestick.

In this way, the character of Simon tells us something about embryonic psychoanalytic technique. However, the insertion of a quasi-analyst into the fictional inquiry into Grace Marks also focuses on the exquisite tension between any nodes of narrative exchange, be they between analysand and analyst, or the teller of a tale and its reader/interpreter. At least initially, Simon has a clear agenda which determines his line of questioning, driven both by the exigencies of Reverend Verringer's employment and his own curiosity to 'attempt, gently and by degrees, to re-establish the chain of thought, which was broken, perhaps by the shock of the violent events in which she was involved'.[11] In other words, Simon's most conscious aim is to solve the riddle of the mysterious woman, to fill in the vital missing gap in Grace's memory, thus conclusively establishing if, and perhaps even why, she committed the crimes. His desire for a particular outcome will of course inevitably influence the process of exchange with Grace, and in addition it is his own largely unacknowledged desires which sabotage his entire ontological project.

The reader is drawn into both positions in this dialectic of exchange: we identify with Grace by means of the first-person voice which Simon elicits and by the very poignancy of much of what she relates—her own narrative of victimisation, naivety and loss. Yet we are also structurally identified with Simon in our own desire and struggle to read the text of Grace—Grace as a historical figure and as a psychology (possibly psychotic) who in turn is necessarily refracted through the imaginative interpretations of the author. In this sense, any act of 'reading' Atwood's narrative of the Grace/Simon exchange graphically demonstrates the ways in which the process is akin to that of psychoanalysis. Not only is it analogous, but because of the very observations of psychoanalytic theory we are invited to read it 'differently'—indeed, in some ways, to operate as an apparently more effective analyst than Simon himself while still, like him, confronting the obstacle of our own desires in the quest for answers or resolution.

By means of the various insights offered by the array of texts which form Atwood's novel, as well as with the help of the formalised methods and ideas developed within psychoanalytic theory since the historical point at which Simon and Grace meet, the reader is seemingly able to proceed further than Simon in an analysis of Grace, her motivations and, less conclusively, her deeds. For instance, although Simon certainly offers her a wider sphere of topics to discuss than she has experienced perhaps ever before, he does fail to fully 'listen' and analyse the myriad of details which she puts before him. Indeed he mistrusts Grace's detailed recollections, missing the opportunity either to read her elaborate narratives as screen memories which might occlude important resistances, or to fully explore their intricacy for large, psychological patterns emergent even in the descriptions of the mundane.

As the analyst/interpreter, Simon, like all readers, is hampered by his own unacknowledged desires and investment in certain kinds of readings or conclusions—in psychoanalytic terms, by his failure to grapple with the complexities of his own position within the gridlock of transference/counter-transference exchange. In particular, his ability to hear the complex nuances, or literally, the different voices within Grace's narratives, is fatally compromised by his desire for personal success in unlocking Grace's mysteries, and perhaps especially by his unacknowledged sexual interest in her. This interest in turn leads to his own playing out of the sexual fantasy with his landlady Rachel Humphrey and the final distraction from his engagement with a text/patient who has become too confronting, whose story has become disturbingly blurred with his own. In this sense, Simon becomes as much a potential instance of the power of repressed or unacknowledged psychic material as Grace, demonstrating through his incipiently violent and erratic behaviour Freud's point that when the 'patient cannot remember the whole of what is repressed in him . . . he is obliged to *repeat* the repressed material as a contemporary experience'.[12]

In contrast to the hubris of Simon as interpreter and reader, Grace at least has a sense of what she *doesn't* know, or what she can't make coherent. In an analogy drawn from her domestic sphere, she speaks of her earliest life in Ireland:

> I don't recall the place very well, as I was a child when I left it; only in scraps, like a plate that's been broken. There are always some pieces that would seem to belong to another plate altogether; and then there are the empty spaces, where you cannot fit anything in.[13]

Piecing together broken crockery, making sense of the patterns of quilts, taking threads and scraps from a variety of places and experiences—all emblematise Grace's efforts to assemble a narrative that makes sense of her life, and particularly of its defining moments of trauma and loss. Focused on the black and white issue of Grace's guilt or innocence of the murders of Nancy and Mr Kinnear, Simon misses both Grace's own attempts at a healing narrative of remembering—as particularly evidenced through the creative artistry of her quilting—and the stray threads or clues which are strewn throughout the narrative which he elicits from her. While Simon hears just the 'usual' tale of poor Irish immigration and struggle,[14] Grace reveals a trail of loss, despair and guilt and complex psychological responses that offer significant insight into whatever violence occurred at Mr Kinnear's house.

As Margaret Rogerson argues, Grace's 'intense interest in patchwork quilts and their designs',[15] both in her own work and that of others, indicates a site of psychological working-through which potentially provides a rich ground for the exploration of her state of mind and motivations. Atwood herself mimics Grace in this as she structures her own narrative of exploration around the cryptic motifs of North American quilt design, organising her chapters around the patterns which conventionally reveal as much as they conceal about the lives of the women who produced them in apparent domestic innocuousness. The graphic designs of the quilts which Grace describes as well as the images which preface Atwood's sections speak volumes for those who pay attention to them, although at the same time their messages are coded and oblique, and reminiscent of Emily Dickinson's exhortation to 'Tell all the Truth but tell it slant—/Success in Circuit Lies'.[16] What is available for speech or narrative is not a pure nub to be extracted, but is both subject to multiple layers of consciousness and fragmentation and necessarily refracted through the very processes of narrative formation.

Using the imagistic tools of the novelist, Atwood herself embroiders Grace's narrative with what may or may not offer clues to her behaviour and the mystery of her mind and motivations. For example at the point of her initial catastrophic loss—the death of her mother on board ship—Grace's feelings of grief and vulnerability are overtaken by a sense of guilt. Having failed to open the window to let out her mother's spirit as advised by a fellow passenger, when a basket containing a precious teapot subsequently falls, the material shattering clearly echoes Grace's emotional state. In what is to emerge as a psychotic connection, her response is to view the breakage as evidence both of her own failings and of the powerful vindictiveness of the dead, creating, through repression or inappropriate mental suturing, what Freud described as 'the appearance of some "daemonic" force at work'.[17] Initiating also the debilitating confusion between her own identity and that of the loved other who betrays her in death, she fearfully relates:

> I thought it was my mother's spirit, trapped in the bottom of the ship because we could not open a window, and angry at me because of the second-best sheet. And now she would be caught in there for ever and ever, down below in the hold like a moth in a bottle, sailing back and forth across the hideous dark ocean, with the emigrants going one way and the logs of wood the other.[18]

This volatile nexus of guilt, grief and rage, caught like an angry 'moth in a bottle', reappears at two crucial times in Grace's narrative. First, it recurs at the point of the death of Mary Whitney. From the almost rapturous description of her life at Mrs Alderman Parkinson's and in particular of her intense, familial friendship with Mary Whitney, there is a sense that healing may yet have been possible for Grace. Still essentially a child, the security and love which she experienced within that household and from Mary in particular seemed to offer a way out of the turmoil of her past—emotional, economic and sexual. There are suggestions in the text that Grace herself was the victim of her father's sexual violence.[19] The death of Mary, directly caused, in Grace's view, by the sexual exploitation of a wealthy, predatory male, reopens Grace's barely healed wounds of loss and vulnerability. She opens the window onto the death bed: 'I was hoping Mary's soul would fly out the window now, and not stay inside, whispering things into my ear. But I wondered whether I was too late'.[20] Immediately afterwards she falls into a swoon of unconsciousness which leaves her confused about her own and Mary's identity, and prefigures the 'alias' of identity which Grace both uses to cope with her situation and yet which eventually dominates and possesses her.

Finally, the night before Nancy and Mr Kinnear are murdered, Mary appears to Grace in a dream—not in a scene from their shared past but, for Grace, 'present' in the very room in which Grace slept with Nancy:

> She was holding a glass tumbler in her hand, and inside it was a firefly, trapped and glowing with a cold and greenish fire. Her face was very pale, but she looked at me and smiled; and then she took her hand from the top of the glass, and the firefly came out and darted about the room; and I knew that this was her soul, and it was trying to find its way out, but the window was shut; and then I could not see where it was gone. Then I woke up, with tears of sadness running down my face, because Mary was lost to me once more.[21]

The challenge of Grace as enigma is also tackled by Dr Jerome DuPont, himself a cryptic character who also operates under a variety of aliases and who, in the form of Jeremiah the pedlar, claims the young Grace into a mysterious fraternity with the comment, 'You are one of us'.[22] As Dr DuPont he tries, where Simon has failed, to elicit the truth from Grace, and gets far more than he bargained for. Using techniques more akin to those of Mesmer and hypnosis, and seemingly operating with Grace as his accomplice in disguise, the experiment ricochets out of his control. The 'voice' which is elicited, which calls itself Mary Whitney, is sarcastic and malevolent—to DuPont and his blatant attempts to predetermine the outcome of his interaction with Grace, to Simon and his erotic innuendoes, to the spiritualists and philanthropists who would redeem the hapless Grace.

In many ways, the episode functions as a shocking moment of revelation in the text, in that we see, or feel we see, that the concept of 'alias' goes well beyond the conscious adoption of disguise to help Grace flee. Rather, her entire identity, or sense of self, has become psychotically and vindictively merged with that of Mary. On one level, 'Mary' has become that aspect of Grace's identity which contains the violent rage, grieving and sense of victimisation which has proved utterly incompatible with her other self; where 'Mary' has acted, in whatever malicious and essentially infantile ways, 'Grace' has been absent, unable to ever recall something she had not done. It is a pivotal textual moment in which the concept of identity in all its myriad complexities apparently flickers into visibility. The narrative appears, retrospectively and prospectively, to fall into comprehensibility. However, Atwood immediately pulls the reader back from such an assumption: we don't in fact know the extent to which DuPont and Grace have colluded in the exercise. As Simon feels, DuPont may just be offering a very reductive and simplistic solution to a far more complex psychological state; DuPont, like Simon, is uncertain and unstable enough as a character for us to question the validity of his finding. We don't for that matter know to what extent Grace herself is consciously in charge of what is ostensibly 'revealed' about her. We can't even, with any surety, dismiss the seemingly ridiculous idea of spiritual 'possession'. What is apparently a conclusion almost immediately dissolves into uncertainty and further questions. The narrative of Grace must continue to unfold and to replay because, by definition, it cannot produce the kernel of truth; it cannot hold the mirror up to identity.

Truth and lies remain inextricably entwined at the close of the novel, much like the ambiguous border which Grace sews into her final Tree of Paradise quilt, which she describes, cryptically and perhaps mischievously, as 'snakes entwined' and yet which she imagines others viewing 'like vines or just a cable pattern'.[23] If, as Rogerson claims, 'This quilt project is Grace's gathering together of the fragments of her life into a whole that is of her own fashioning'—after a lifetime in which others have written or ghosted the scripts which defined her—it is a 'whole which remains mysterious . . .

Does the quilt represent memory, amnesia or madness?'[24] Grace herself continues the business of revelation and concealment and Atwood closes the novel by allowing the narrative's view to be largely aligned with her first-person thoughts. And though there are significant breaks with the past suggested by Grace's release from incarceration—her reconciliation with the formerly betraying Jamie Walsh, and even her geographical move back 'across the lake' to the United States—the narrative also clearly stresses the impossibility of starting anew, of completely severing the cords which bind an individual to the past.

Grace *may* have made significant advances on a path to acceptance or integration of her past—or she may not have, just as she doesn't know if what is growing within her belly is a 'life or a death'.[25] The final image of the quilt (in many ways a long-deferred response to Simon's question about apples), graphically inscribes the fundamental questions which remain. It is a work of art which can be seen to narrate, to gather up and to recollect what had arguably previously only been compulsively repeated. Grace's careful stitching places together, at least in a semblance of closure, her personal points of intensity and trauma—reconnecting fragments of the petticoat from Mary Whitney, a prison nightdress, and Nancy's 'pink and white floral' so that 'we will all be together'.[26] It *may* be an image of healing, of integration rather than repression. Or, chillingly, it may yet be acknowledgment of the continuing presence and pressure of the past, for better *or* worse.

Like the narratives of psychoanalysis, the literary narrative produced by Atwood portrays an identity that is problematic and necessarily fractured. While the identity of Grace Marks is highlighted and apparently exceptional due to the violence of the crimes and the mystery adhering to the beautiful young maidservant, in fact the exceptional instance simply serves to emphasise the elusiveness of any conclusive narrative about the self. In a quest for knowledge and epistemological certainty, we as readers come armed with sets of strategies such as historical reference, external forms of verification, textual and psychological examination and of course personal interpretation in order to attempt to chisel free the identity of the novel's central character, to arrive at the answer to whatever puzzle or absence the narrative might be predicated upon. Inevitably, as for Simon, that task fails because its premises are flawed. Despite the most compelling of narrative presentations, identity or subjectivity will always remain episodic and riddled with contradiction; and as a text like Atwood's exposes, such an epistemological quest reveals as much about our own desire for control over the external world as it does about exteriority itself.

In his essay 'Structure, Sign, and Play', Jacques Derrida identifies this schism in the nature of any act of textual interpretation, which in turn is integrally linked to the production of text itself:

There are thus two interpretations of interpretation, of structure, of sign, of play. The one seeks to decipher, dreams of deciphering, a truth or an origin which escapes play and the order of the sign, and which lives the necessity of interpretation as an exile. The other, which is no longer turned toward the origin, affirms play and tries to pass beyond man and humanism, the name of man being the name of the being who . . . has dreamed of full presence, the reassuring foundation, the origin and the end of play.[27]

Alias Grace demonstrates the persistence of both modes of interpretation in reading the conundrum of identity. It reaffirms our desire to know and define the concept of subjectivity almost despite the impossibility of doing so, despite repeated rebuffs and collapses into the chaos of what Derrida ironically calls the 'order of the sign'. Mystery would appear to be the origin around which such concepts of interpretation revolve. But it is a hollow and ironic centre which returns both the reader and the subject marked by such mystery to the play of narratives—partial narratives that offer episodic or imagistic insights into the subject and its circumstances, and narratives that are interminably retold and reshaped and which, in their telling, perhaps come closest to constructing the shifting palimpsest of identity.

Conclusion: politics, history and the unconscious

John Cash

IN *THE CEMENT OF SOCIETY* Jon Elster comments, regarding the Swedish system of collective bargaining, that a detailed study of this 'moving, fluid process' of collective bargaining forced him to recognise that 'everything is up for grabs: the identities of the actors, the rules of the game, the set of payoffs, the range of acceptable arguments.'[1] It seems to me that this statement might be made just as readily about all social and political processes: that all such processes are (potentially) dynamic as regards the characteristics of the subjects in interaction, as regards the rules and reasons which organise the process, and consequentially as regards the characteristics of what counts as an interest and a reward. In other words, and now these are my words, between them ideology and subjectivity constitute the dynamic field upon which social and political processes are enacted and in terms of which interests are calculated and reasons are evaluated.

Next let me quote from Jessica Benjamin's *The Bonds of Love*:

At times we [feminists] are shocked by how much the reality of woman's condition differs from what we, in our minds, have long since determined it should be. Even the more modest demands for equality that we take for granted have not been realised. So it was when two psychologists, one of them the mother of a newborn boy, strolled by the hospital nursery to peer through the glass at the other newborns. Of course each bassinet had a pink or blue label proclaiming the swaddled baby's sex, which would otherwise be indecipherable (what confusion might that bring!). But astonishment overcame them when they looked at the first pink label. Expecting to find the counterpart to the blue one, which proudly announced, 'I'm a boy!' they found instead, 'It's a girl!' Further examination forced them to confirm what they at first refused to believe: all the boys were 'I' and all the girls were 'It.' The infant girl was already presented to the world not as a potential 'I,' but as an object, 'It.' The sexual difference was already interpreted in terms of complementary and unequal roles, subject and object. The aspect of will, desire, and activity—all that we might conjure up with a subject who is an 'I'—was assigned to the male gender alone.[2]

What I would like to add to this, though not by way of contradicting Benjamin, is the point that each of us, male or female, as we grow from infancy to adulthood, is caught between the force and attraction of that nameless 'It' and the fragile pretension of the shifting, though persevering, 'I'. Each of us, unless we go 'mad', finds a dynamic accommodation between the It and the I, an accommodation which, though it tends to persist, is constantly reworked within the moving field of rules, reasons and emotions which we can denote as culture or ideology. In other words, as subjects we are doubly decentred. The shifting though persevering I which we each take ourself to be is always subject to reorganisation according to the rules of the It, or more precisely, the dynamic unconscious. This is its first decentring. At the same time this same shifting, though persevering, I is subject to reorganisation according to the rules of the field of ideology. This is the second moment of its decentring. These two moments of decentring are, of course, each implicated in the other. Between them they constitute both the bases of subjection and, although it might at first appear paradoxical, the grounds of agency and of the subject's partial penetration of those processes (both psychic and ideological) which determine the character of his or her very subjectivity. Together these two moments of decentring constitute both the limits to, as well as the potentialities for, agency, reason, individuality and solidarity. In their referencing of the subjective and the social, they draw together the key terms of our current concerns: politics and history on the one hand, and the unconscious on the other. It is as decentred subjects—doubly decentred, as I am suggesting—that we find our place and take our place in the ongoing history of the present and in the politics through which this historical process is shaped.

So in what follows I want to lay out the bare bones of an argument that attempts to draw together our key terms: history and the unconscious. In particular I want to try to outline an approach which joins these two terms in a way that opens onto an analysis of the political, rather than operating in a manner that forecloses the political—which ironically is usually the case.

Anyone who is well acquainted with Freud's case studies is inevitably well aware of the intricate, delicate, complex and over-determined imbrication of history and the unconscious that is narrated and analysed in them. At every turn, the history of the subject (including a dynamic 'archaeology' and 'genealogy' of the subject)—a history that is both continuous and discontinuous, familiar and surprising, hence always uncanny—is deepened and extended through the techniques and concepts of psychoanalytic practice. This history, then—a history of events, experiences, and constructions and a history of the memories and fantasies attached to such events, experiences, and constructions—is reconstructed and retold through close attention to the unconscious with its various processes and formations. In the hands of a writer such as Freud or Klein, there is no disjunction between a focus on the unconscious and the retelling of a life—a retelling that holds out the prospect of a remaking of a life. An adequate history of the subject inevitably entails entering into the confounding complexities of an uncanny unconscious. Richard Rorty makes a similar point very nicely in his essay 'The Contingency of Selfhood' when he writes:

> For Freud, nobody is dull through and through, for there is no such thing as a dull unconscious. What makes Freud more useful and more plausible than Nietzsche is that he does not relegate the vast majority of humanity to the status of dying animals. For Freud's account of unconscious fantasy shows us how to see every human life as a poem . . .[3]

In suggesting this Rorty is highlighting the manner in which Freud's invention of psychoanalysis enabled a profound extension and deepening of our abilities to retell the history of a life, in all its canny and uncanny dimensions.

This imbrication of history and the unconscious is also a feature of social relations that stretch beyond the purview and scope of an individual life. But in this arena the couplet of history and the unconscious is a less happy and productive one. We might say that a bar has inserted itself between the terms of the couplet: the bar of the social. This bar unsettles and undercuts the creative potential of the couplet, tending to generate a flattening-out of complexity and a narrowed, one-dimensional account of history as a repetition compulsion. In what follows I will try to explain why this happens, illustrate the characteristic forms it takes and finally briefly outline an approach that overcomes these characteristic limitations.

Where psychoanalysis and history join hands in the reconstruction of an individual life or in the exploration of a group experience, the best practitioners of the art address the contingent effects of social process (and specific, often traumatic, events), by analysing the ways in which such processes and events mark themselves upon the subject. These marks—as the poet William Blake[4] would term them—sometimes recognised by the subject, more often misrecognised or unrecognised, attach themselves to and shape what I previously termed a history of events, experiences, and constructions and a history of the memories and fantasies attached to them. As

Rorty has noted, they are what another poet, Philip Larkin, has termed 'the blind impress/All our behavings bear'.[5]

Such exemplary studies, by foregrounding the synthetic registration and reconstitution of contingent historical processes and events within the experience and within the knowing/unknowingness of the subject, bring into focus the full realm of history and the unconscious as they intersect, overlap and over-determine the history of the subject. The knowing/unknowingness of the subject provides the horizon within which interpretation and analysis can proceed.

There is a cost, or at least a limit, to such an approach. This limit is neared as analytic attention shifts from the study of an individual or a specific grouping with a common and for the moment shared identity, towards the analysis of larger groupings, more complex institutions and whole societies. At some point along this continuum it becomes necessary to pull back from an immersion in the imaginary identifications and symbolic anchorings of an individual or group and attempt to more systematically theorise social processes and their 'blind impress' upon doubly decentred subjects. This is where the difficulties begin; it is in executing this move that a flattening-out of experience, memory and fantasy is typically produced. Dennis Wrong is correct in suggesting that it is here that the 'oversocialised conception of man' has left *its* dulling impress.[6]

As Wrong indicates, the 'most fundamental insight' of psychoanalysis is 'that the wish, the emotion and the fantasy are as important as the act in man's experience'.[7] (We might catch an implied reference to Blake here). However, this complexity of thought and feeling, fantasy and desire, typically is screened out in those very instances where attempts are made to systematically introduce a theory that addresses the intersection of social processes and the unconscious. This occurs because most sociology and social theory has appropriated psychoanalysis as a theory of socialisation. This psychoanalytically inflected socialisation theory has cast a long, dark shadow upon a multitude of empirical studies that turn to psychoanalysis for a better conceptualisation of subjectivity. The shadow of socialisation has fallen upon the subject (and his or her connection to the social and the political), we might say. The result has been a long melancholia of distorted understandings about the internal relations of our couplet of history and the unconscious.

Let me take the classic example of the Frankfurt School. In this tradition psychoanalysis was turned to in order to better understand the dialectic of the Enlightenment, in particular in order to reveal and analyse the dark underside of the Enlightenment project. Psychoanalysis was characterised as a materialist science that could explain the ways in which ideology operated as a social cement that stabilised and naturalised (that is, rendered proper and natural) prevailing class relations. The key to all this lay in the crucible of the family, the critical institution within which socialisation proceeded. It was in the family, understood as a historically specific and hence variable institution, that the functional requirements of the economy secured themselves and found their guarantee within the personality structure of the individual subject. For monopoly capital, the specific family culture functional for the reproduction of the society was of a sadomasochistic type—hence the new anthropological type nurtured by monopoly capital was the authoritarian personality. As Erich Fromm put it: 'The family is the medium through which the society or the social class stamps its specific structure on the child, and hence on the adult. The family is the psychological agency of society'.[8]

In this move something is gained—an ability to characterise the typical pattern of desire within a population. We might say that a certain historical specificity is introduced via this apparent gain. But much more is lost. The subject is reduced to a mere marker and repository of the system logic, now described in psychoanalytic terms. Perhaps more significantly, history—as a contingent process that is made and remade in the recurrent here and now of an unfolding social process—is eclipsed. It is reduced to the repetition of a trait-like attribute that oddly centres the subject, along with all the neighbours and strangers within that society. Once established, this character trait is set as a libidinal organisation, or personality structure, that persists and cements the subject into his or her place within the social order. This is achieved through ideology that at once reiterates the system logic (the functional requirements of monopoly capital) and satisfies the desires of the authoritarian type (the modal personality of the time).

It is perhaps worth noting that a similar argument is deployed by Daniel Goldhagen in *Hitler's Willing Executioners*. While avoiding psychoanalytic concepts, Goldhagen relies implicitly on a socialisation argument in which a common cultural code, 'eliminationist antisemitism', becomes an internalised attribute of virtually all German citizens—it becomes part of their 'cognitive model', in his terminology. Hence, in discussing the relationship between German culture and the German citizen, Goldhagen argues that the cognitive model of eliminationist anti-Semitism 'is incorporated into the structures of his mind as naturally as the grammar of his language', as he puts it.[9] Goldhagen is quite explicit about characterising this cognitive model as the 'independent' variable that, of itself, operated as the motivational cause of the Holocaust.[10] Other contingencies, such as the rise to power of the Nazi party, played a part, but the motivation to participate willingly in the extermination of the Jews is explained via a rather cursory socialisation model. The effect of this is to characterise the Holocaust as a kind of dreadful appointment just waiting to happen, due to the persistence, over a lengthy historical period of a stable disposition: the common orientation of most Germans towards the elimination and extermination of Jews.

Goldhagen's bold thesis helps us to see the limits of any approach to social relations that relies unduly on socialisation assumptions and on the related assumption of human subjects as psychologically centred in a particular pattern of belief. Such an approach overstates the supposedly fixed centredness of certain dispositions and beliefs and systematically screens out the ways in which these remain open to modification and reorganisation in the unfolding here and now of historical contingency and conflict. In the process such an approach risks dehumanising whole populations by ascribing to them prejudices or, as in this case, deadly motivations that are taken to be fixed, intrinsic aspects of their internal psychic structure. Ironically, the very mentality that is repudiated by the analysis, as in Goldhagen, resurfaces in the account that is developed about the national character under consideration.

Perhaps I have now stated enough to make it clear why I have addressed Goldhagen's work in this context. The mention of national character above should alert us to a hidden, perhaps repressed, lineage of analysis and interpretation that lies behind Goldhagen's work, and yet it has never been acknowledged, nor even identified, so far as I am aware. This lineage is of course that long tradition of national character analysis that stretches back into the founding moments of an intersection between psychoanalysis and the writing of sociology and history, a moment that began to define itself soon after World War II. The classic example of this genre is Erik Erikson's *Childhood and Society*, in which he links culturally specific socialisation experiences to prevalent subjective orientations. Socialisation is understood as producing a particular personality disposition which, once established, subsequently plays a major role in determining behaviour.

Another classic in this genre is the study conducted by Henry Dicks during World War II and subsequently published as 'Personality Traits and National Socialist Ideology'. In this subtle study Dicks registers the kind of qualification that Goldhagen would have been wise to follow, when he suggests that it 'is not the intention in these pages to pillory the German people' and explains that he does 'not assert that such traits [of national character] are found in equal degree, or at all, in all members of that group, or that they are so conjoined that the extreme is also the norm'.[11] However, despite these qualifications, the basic premise remains problematic. By attributing so much causal independence to an internal psychic state, itself understood as the product of a culturally characteristic socialisation process, the analysis of social and historical processes is unduly weighted towards an emphasis on supposedly stable, internal psychic preconditions of whole populations and directed away from a focus on the myriad social and political conflicts of the contemporary moment. In effect the human subject is centred and frozen in his or her culturally specific prejudice or pattern of motivation and historical explanation is reduced to a sifting-through of factors that either facilitate or obstruct the acting out of the internalised and stabilised model or trait. While avoiding any mention of its repressed psychoanalytic heritage, Goldhagen's work is exemplary in the way it provides a contemporary illustration of the profound limitations of the socialisation model of writing politics and history. This said, there is, indeed, an oddly revealing way in which this repressed psychoanalytic heritage returns within Goldhagen's study. In several places he characterises German constructions of Jews as 'hallucinatory'.[12]

Another classic study of the pivotal role played by socialisation in the preparation for, or inoculation against, fascism is of course *The Authoritarian Personality*. I mention this by way of introducing some reflections on a heterodox follow-up to *The Authoritarian Personality* written by Theodor Adorno in 1951. In 'Freudian Theory and the Pattern of Fascist Propaganda' Adorno presents a far more complex account of the social and psychic processes through which fascism might spread, than anything that is anticipated in the multi-authored study of authoritarianism. My own understanding of this article is that it served a defensive purpose for Adorno; it was a means by which Adorno distanced himself from the rather awkward methodological individualism of *The Authoritarian Personality*, with its exaggerated focus on the socialised individual actor or subject and its corresponding adoption of a psychoanalytically inflected socialisation model. Adorno begins his 1951 article by turning to Freud's 'Group Psychology and the Analysis of the Ego'.[13] In doing so he sidesteps the characteristic emphasis on socialisation and opens onto the processes of identification that support the emergence of a group mentality in the here and now of the historical present. In this way Adorno catches the doubly decentred character of subjectivity as it is conceptualised by Freud in 'Group Psychology and the Analysis of the Ego'.

In Louis Althusser's 'Ideology and the Ideological State Apparatuses' essay we see an instance of a major break with the socialisation argument.[14] And yet even here in the little quasi-empirical examples of the communications and educational state apparatuses, the ghost of the socialisation thesis survives. It is there in the notion that the communications apparatus operates by 'cramming every citizen with daily doses of nationalism', and in the notion that the education apparatus 'drums into them ... a certain amount of know-how wrapped in the ruling ideology'.[15] Of course, in the latter part of the essay, in his more structuralist account of ideology in general, of ideology that has no history, Althusser makes a paradigmatic break that enables him to treat ideology as 'a new reality', as he puts it.[16] While this move—a move towards a theory of interpellation as the dynamic moment in which history and the unconscious intersect in the making of a particular, historical subject—opened up a whole new domain of inquiry, in Althusser's own hands it quickly collapsed back into a neo-functionalism in which the complex particularity of any specific ideological formation was read through the rigid grid of its function within the reproduction of the conditions of production. At once the intersection of history and the unconscious was both radically reconceptualised and chronically reduced.

It is my own sense that a parallel phenomenon can be seen in Slavoj Zizek's work. I think it is now clear that Zizek's work plays out in much more detail, and in a register that is more concerned with the Lacanian conceptualisation of the real, a similar trajectory to Althusser's. For all his brilliance, what I find unsatisfactory about Zizek's joining of psychoanalysis and a history of the present is the way in which he constantly returns to the basic ontological question of subjectivity—the so-called ticklish subject—and plays out the general argument about the need to suture or mend the gap in the symbolic order, to cover over the fact that the big Other doesn't exist. This draws him away from a systematic exploration and analysis of specific fantasy structures, of specific ideologies and the ways in which they operate to organise or structure social relations. Of course he routinely discusses a variety of fantasy structures at some length, but mainly this discussion reiterates the general claim about how such fantasy structures cover over the fact that the big Other doesn't exist.

What we don't get is the kind of detailed attention to the way a particular fantasy structure organises the subject in a particular way over time, as in the Freud case studies. Nor do we get the close attention to the unconscious structures that organise subjective and social experience, that organise intersubjectivity and the culture of institutions, as in the case studies of such writers as Elliott Jacques and Isabel Menzies from within the Tavistock tradition. For all its theoretical limitations, in this Kleinian-derived approach the emphasis is on finding out something particular about how a specific institution with a historically specific cultural defence mechanism works—there is an opening onto historical and political specificity. Zizek gives us very little of this. We hear about several fantasy structures in *The Ticklish Subject*, for instance, but mainly we hear about how they operate to depoliticise the economy by regarding it as a given, as a kind of natural fact that cannot be altered. Such ideologies blind us to the possibility of ordering our societies differently and fascinate us with less significant issues. So racism, sexism, nationalism, globalism, consumerism and the multifarious other ideologies through which identities are organised and performed are collapsed back into so many layers over a primary antagonism that circulates through the international capitalist economy, and yet can never be named and opposed for what it is. As I understand it, this removes the decentred subject, the ticklish subject, from any capacity for historical agency. Indeed it ontologises the bar between history and the unconscious, effectively removing the subject from the knowing/unknowing making of history. Politics as anything other than the play of disciplinary power are eclipsed—and of course in that move the very logic of addressing the interplay of politics, history and the unconscious is similarly eclipsed. It is a strange position for this approach to end up in—and a rather uncanny return to Althusser's blind spot.

This, then, is the dilemma. Typically the conjoining of history and the unconscious through some version of a socialisation model flattens out the dynamic complexity of the human subject by reducing this subject to a specific identification which is taken to be both socially (or economically) functional and quite stable. Identity, then, becomes a fixed identity produced as an effect of some systemic requirement. Of course this generates an account in which historicity is disavowed. What is not observed in this approach is the very stuff of history: the conflicted, contested, dynamic making and remaking of identity and social relations in the contingent here and now and an ongoing psychic process of identification that leans on culture and the social in their multiplicity. It is in this leaning upon culture and the social that history and the unconscious are joined. This is never a once-and-for-all settling of an identity. Rather it is an ongoing process in which, for the moment, a particular identification seems to constitute an essence worth preserving and fighting over. At another moment this same identification may shift or be displaced, sometimes after intense conflict.

This fraught contestation over shifting identifications is better grasped through conceptualisations that are open to the dynamics of a ticklish subject in process. However, the characteristic approach of this type, in a tradition stretching from A to Z so to speak (from Althusser to Zizek), involves disarticulating the ontological amorphousness of the subject from the conditioning and marking effects of the historically specific culture and society, thereby either reifying or occluding the political. The very structure of Althusser's argument in his 'Ideology and the Ideological State Apparatuses' essay, which so readily falls into the part of history and the part of the unconscious, bears exquisite witness to this division.

I have already suggested above that the ghost of the socialisation argument returns to the very place from which it has been evicted when Althusser fudges the leaning of history upon the unconscious via a crude socialisation argument of an entirely functionalist kind. Zizek does not do this. Rather, through a habit of attention that moves between anecdote and ontology and keeps reasserting the inherent failure of identification, Zizek effectively disregards the significance of the social and political processes through which specific identifications are established for the moment. He also puts aside the subsequent effectiveness of these very identifications as they consolidate themselves and become the moment of subjective organisation from within which history is made again and anew, both knowingly and unknowingly. Ironically Zizek can find no way of incorporating the relative autonomy of a specific ideology into an account of the leaning of history upon the unconscious. The dilemma, then, is that accounts of subjectivity typically vacillate between a foreclosing of the radical openness of subjectivity, as in the socialisation model, and a disavowal of the power (the invested effectivity) of contingently formed, yet for the moment organised, particular subjectivities. How might such a vicious circle be squared?

The approach I advocate, and have developed elsewhere, is a radically extended theory of structuration that directly addresses the structuration of the unconscious within culture and society. Such an approach begins with a depth hermeneutics of the unconscious rules, or imaginaries, that organise patterns of identity and intersubjectivity in a specific historical setting. The particular case I have focused upon most is Northern Ireland. But the same issues arise in conceptualising cases such as Australian nationalism or America's response(s) to September 11.

Already, in 'Group Psychology and the Analysis of the Ego', Freud addressed the ways in which contingent processes in the here and now of both institutional and psychic life leaned in upon each other and took particular form through processes of identification. A group mentality with specific features took form, itself the product of either emergent or (in 'artificial' groups such as the army or the church) established unconscious rules. Freud's approach runs quite counter to the socialisation model because it keeps open and contingent the organisation of subjectivity, which is always a subjectivity established out of contestation and conflict and stabilised only for the moment—even if, in cases of deeply entrenched social institutions, this moment is a lengthy one.

By extension we can see that ideologies or discourses, and in particular their unconscious rules or imaginaries, are central to social and political life because they establish, through processes of identification and internalisation, the range of common-sense understandings, the predominant reality principles, that are recursively drawn upon by subjects to construe how to be and how to act. At the same time what counts as proper—the proper way of being, relating, feeling or construing—is recurrently fought over in the ongoing making and remaking of social and political relations. These unconscious rules, in their multiple codings of the proper, including the proper form of authority, the proper exercise of power and the proper form of violence, become the very object over which a politics of identity is played out. At issue is which set of unconscious rules, each with quite distinct and conflicting implications for the organisation of identities and social relations, will become predominant for the moment.

In such an approach the internal forms of any ideology or fantasy structure are analysed more for what they produce than for what they occlude. The emphasis falls on the positivity and performativity of any specific ideology or imaginary. This draws attention to the making and remaking of particular formations of the unconscious within a social and cultural organisation or institution. It brings into focus the patterns of thinking, feeling, reasoning and relating that come to constitute particular forms of common sense and the particular discourses through which identities are organised and reorganised in the intended and unintended making of the present. Thereby it reintroduces politics into the couplet—history and the unconscious.

Notes

Abbreviations

ANRC	Australian National Research Council
CITF	Civilian Internees Trust Fund
DFT	Donald Thomson Papers, NAA
DT	Donald Thomson Private Papers
NAA	National Archives of Australia
NLA	National Library of Australia
SLV	State Library of Victoria
VPRS	Victorian Public Records Series

Introduction: psychoanalysis, histories and identities

[1] Schwartz, *Cassandra's Daughter*, p. 1.
[2] de Certeau, *Heterologies*, pp. 1–4.
[3] Gay, *Freud for Historians*, p. 3.
[4] ibid., pp. 3–4.
[5] ibid., p. 119.
[6] Gay, *The Naked Heart*, p. 8.
[7] ibid., p. 3.
[8] ibid., p. 10.
[9] ibid., p. 9.
[10] Roper, *Oedipus and the Devil*, p. 8.
[11] ibid., pp. 26–7.
[12] Alexander, 'Feminist History and Psychoanalysis', in *Becoming a Woman*, pp. 225–6.
[13] ibid., p. 229.
[14] Davidoff, 'Class and Gender in Victorian England', pp. 103–50, 206–26.
[15] Jan Lewis and Peter N. Stearns, 'Introduction', in *An Emotional History of the United States*, pp. 6–7.
[16] Steele, 'The Gender and Racial Politics of Mourning in Antebellum America', pp. 91–106.
[17] Gergen, 'History and Psychology', pp. 15–29.
[18] Figlio, 'Historical Imagination/Psychoanalytic Imagination', pp. 199–221.
[19] de Certeau, *Heterologies*.
[20] Pick, 'Freud's Group Psychology and the History of the Crowd', pp. 30–61.
[21] Altman, *Global Sex*.

[22] See Caruth, *Trauma*; Tal, *World of Hurt*; Antze and Lambeck, *Tense Past*; LaCapra, *History and Memory After Auschwitz*.

[23] Caruth, *Trauma*, pp. 4–5.

[24] Phillips, *Promises, Promises*, p. 41.

[25] Jackson, *Literature, Psychoanalysis and the New Sciences of the Mind*.

[26] Hunt, 'No Longer an Evenly Flowing River', pp. 1517–21.

1 Hearing the 'speech of the excluded'

[1] Alexander, 'Women, Class and Sexual Difference in the 1830s and '40s', published as 'Women, Class and Sexual Difference', in *Becoming a Woman*, pp. 97–125.

[2] Alexander, 'Freud and Psychohistory', in Green and Troup, *The Houses of History*, pp. 59–70; Alexander, 'Women, Class and Sexual Difference', in *Becoming a Woman*, p. 109.

[3] Mills, *Madness, Cannabis and Colonialism*, pp. 21–6.

[4] See Mary Elene Wood, *The Writing on the Wall: Women's Autobiography and the Asylum*, University of Illinois Press, Urbana, Ill., 1994; Jeffrey Geller and Maxine Harris (eds), *Women of the Asylum: Voices from Behind the Walls, 1840–1945*, Anchor Books Doubleday, New York, 1994.

[5] Bronwyn Labrum, 'Looking beyond the Asylum: Gender and the Process of Committal in Auckland, 1870–1910', *The New Zealand Journal of History*, vol. 26, 1992, pp. 125–44.

[6] Anne Catherine Currie, Farm Diaries. See Tony Dingle, 'Anne Currie: Towards a Biography', *Gippsland Heritage Journal*, vol. 1, 1986, pp. 9–13; Shane Carmody, 'The Currie Family in 1888', *Australia 1888 Bulletin*, no. 11, 1983, pp. 32–6; Janice Chesters, 'A Horror of the Asylum or of the Home? Women's Responses to Asylum Confinement', in Catharine Coleborne and Dolly MacKinnon (eds), *'Madness' in Australia: Histories, Heritage and the Asylum*, University of Queensland Press, Brisbane, in press; McLeary, *Catherine*.

[7] valentine, The Making of Modern Madness, ch. 2.

[8] John E. Toews, 'Foucault and the Freudian Subject: Archaeology, Genealogy, and the Historicization of Psychoanalysis', in Goldstein, *Foucault and the Writing of History*, pp. 122, 131–2. See also valentine, The Making of Modern Madness, ch. 2.

[9] Blackman, 'What Is Doing History?', pp. 488–9.

[10] Rose, *Inventing Ourselves*, pp. 26, 107, 114.

[11] Lunbeck, *The Psychiatric Persuasion*, pp. 4, 327n.

[12] ibid., p. 4.

[13] Nikolas Rose, 'Of Madness Itself: *Histoire de la folie* and the Object of Psychiatric History', in Still and Velody, *Rewriting the History of Madness*, pp. 143–5.

[14] 'Religious Mania' and 'Suicide of a Young Woman', the *Age*, 18 September 1883, p. 6.

[15] Margaret Maria M., 4 March 1874, VPRS 7397/P1, Kew Asylum, Unit 2, p. 99.

[16] Helen W., 25 November 1864, VPRS 7400/P1, Yarra Bend Asylum, Unit 2, p. 12.

[17] Charlotte Elizabeth G., 28 July 1870, VPRS 7400/P1, Yarra Bend Asylum, Unit 4, p. 17.

[18] 'Two Cases of Mania', *Australian Medical Journal*, vol. 11, 1866, pp. 197–9.

[19] Weiner, 'Esquirol's Patient Register'.

[20] Burnham, 'Psychoanalysis and American Medicine', pp. 88–9; Mills, *Madness, Cannabis and Colonialism*, p. 5.

[21] Catharine Coleborne, '"She Does up Her Hair Fantastically": The Production of Femininity in Patient Case-books of the Lunatic Asylum in 1860s Victoria', in Helen Brash et al. (eds), *Forging Identities: Bodies, Gender and Feminist History*, University of Western Australia Press, Nedlands, WA, 1997, pp. 47–68.

[22] McLeary, *Catherine*, pp. 85–6.

[23] See also McLeary, *Catherine*, pp. 86–91.

[24] (Anne) Catherine Currie, 17 September 1881, VPRS 7400/P1, Yarra Bend Asylum, Unit 6, p. 331.

[25] Micale, 'Paradigm and Ideology in Psychiatric History Writing', pp. 150–1.

[26] Lunbeck, *The Psychiatric Persuasion*, pp. 23–4.

[27] Burnham, 'Psychoanalysis and American Medicine', pp. 81–2.

28 Philip Cushman, 'Psychotherapy to 1992: A Historically Situated Interpretation', in Free-dheim, *History of Psychotherapy*, pp. 21–64. See also Cushman, *Constructing the Self*.

29 For instance Andrew Scull, *Museums of Madness: The Social Organisation of Insanity in Nineteenth-century England*, Allen Lane, London, 1979, p. 258; Elaine Showalter, *The Female Malady: Women, Madness and English Culture 1830–1980*, Pantheon, New York, 1985, p. 164.

30 Sigmund Freud, 'Psychoanalysis and Psychiatry', Lecture 16, 1916–1917, in *Introductory Lectures on Psychoanalysis*, ed. James Strachey and Angela Richards, trans. James Strachey, Pelican, London, 1974.

31 Stephen Garton, *Medicine and Madness: A Social History of Insanity in New South Wales, 1880–1940*, UNSW Press, Sydney, 1988, p. 82.

32 Currie, Farm Diaries vol. 2, 14 December 1880; any gaps or errors in transcription are my own.

33 ibid., 12 February 1880.

34 *Warragul Guardian*, 22 September 1881, p. 2.

35 Currie, Farm Diaries, vol. 2, 20 September 1881.

36 ibid., 9 October 1881.

37 ibid., October 1881.

38 ibid., 20 October 1881.

39 ibid., 24 January 1882.

40 ibid., October 1881.

41 Lunbeck, *The Psychiatric Persuasion*, pp. 130–3.

42 ibid., p. 4.

43 Foucault, 'Madness, the Absence of Work', pp. 290–1.

44 Comment regarding patient Elizabeth W., 19 March 1869, VPRS 7401/P1, Ararat Asylum, Unit 1, 1867–71, p. 79.

45 Currie, Farm Diaries, 1 January 1894, cited in McLeary, *Catherine*, p. 144; 17 February 1897, p. 159 (emphasis in the original).

46 Porter, *A Social History of Madness*, p. 1.

2 A history of dreams

1 Letter from Reverend J. Leighton-Edwell to Bishop Burgmann, 22 March 1938, Burgmann Papers, box 10, correspondence, 'Psychology'.

2 Letter from Miss A. Frost to Bishop Burgmann, 15 May 1939, ibid.

3 Stephen Garton, 'Freud and the Psychiatrists: The Australian Debate 1900–1940' in Brian Head and James Walter (eds), *Intellectual Movements and Australian Society*, Oxford University Press, Melbourne, 1988, pp. 170–87; Stephen Garton, 'The Melancholy Years: Psychiatry in New South Wales, 1900–1930', in Richard Kennedy (ed.), *Australian Welfare History: Critical Essays*, Macmillan, Sydney, 1982, pp. 138–66; Stephen Garton, 'Freud Versus the Rat: Under-standing Shell Shock in World War I', *Intellect and Emotion: Australian Cultural History*, no. 16, 1997/1998, pp. 45–59.

4 Phillips, *Terrors and Experts*, p. 73.

5 Brett, 'Psychoanalysis in Australia', p. 340.

6 Debra Morris, 'Privacy, Privation and Perversity: Toward New Representations of the Personal', *Signs*, vol. 25, no. 2, Winter 2000, p. 324.

7 White, *Inventing Australia*, pp. 128, 130–5.

8 ibid., p. 155.

9 See Kay Saunders and Raymond Evans (eds), *Gender Relations in Australia: Domination and Negotiation*, Harcourt/Brace/Jovanovich, Sydney, 1990.

10 Rickard, *A Family Romance*.

11 Stuart Macinytre, *The Reds: The Communist Party of Australia, From Origins To Illegality*, Allen & Unwin, Sydney, 1998, pp. 194, 270, 304.

12 Ernest Burgmann, 'The Place of Psychology in Religion', November 1921, pp. 15, 28, Burg-mann Papers, box 20, file 1.

13 ibid., p. 20.

14 Stephen Garton, 'Roy Coupland Winn', *Australian Dictionary of Biography*, vol. 12, Melbourne University Press, Melbourne, pp. 540–1.

15 R. Coupland Winn, 'Psychoanalysis and Allied Forms of Psychotherapy', *Medical Journal of Australia*, 16 November 1940, p. 511.

16 R. Coupland Winn, 'Psychology in Relation to Modern Medical Practice', *Medical Journal of Australia*, 6 December 1930, pp. 752–8.

17 ibid., p. 753.

18 R. Coupland Winn, 'Psycho-analysis in War-time', *Australasian Nurses' Journal*, vol. 15, January 1943, p. 4.

19 Richard Lindstrom, The Australian Experience of Psychological Casualties in War 1915–1939, PhD, Victorian University of Technology, 1997, p. 257.

20 See Rosemary Pringle, *Sex and Medicine: Gender, Power and Authority in the Medical Profession*, Cambridge University Press, Melbourne, 1996, pp. 144–55.

21 See Nellie L. Thompson, 'Early Women Psychoanalysts', *International Review of Psycho-Analysis*, vol. 14, 1987, pp. 397–401.

22 ibid., p. 404.

23 Clive and Neild, 'Utilitarian Education—or The Good Life', *Angry Penguins*, December 1944, pp. 49–51.

24 Curthoys, 'Eugenics, Feminism, and Birth Control', p. 78.

25 Piddington, *Tell Them!*, p. 14.

26 Marion Piddington, 'The Frustration of the Maternal Instinct and the New Psychology', *Australasian Journal of Psychology and Philosophy*, vol. XV, 1937, p. 210.

27 ibid., p. 209.

28 Juliet Mitchell, 'Introduction to Melanie Klein', in Lyndsey Stonebridge and John Phillips (eds), *Reading Melanie Klein*, Routledge, London, 1998, p. 15.

29 *Everylady's Journal*, 1 January 1927, p. 54.

30 ibid., 2 June 1930, p. 542.

31 *Women's World*, 1 August 1926, p. 529.

32 *Everylady's Journal*, 1 July 1926, p. 69.

33 ibid., 1 October 1926, p. 339.

34 Freud, *The Interpretation of Dreams*, pp. 383–453.

35 Ernest Burgmann, Diary 1922, entry 6 March 1922, Burgmann Papers, box 41.

36 Heather Goodall, *Invasion to Embassy: Land in Aboriginal Politics in New South Wales, 1770–1972*, Allen & Unwin, Sydney, 1996, pp. 2–6.

37 Wolfe, 'On Being Woken Up', pp. 206, 210.

38 A. P. Elkin, 'Notes on the Psychic Life of the Australian Aborigines', *Mankind*, vol. 2, no. 3, January 1937, p. 51.

39 Dipesh Chakrabarty, *Provincializing Europe: Postcolonial Thought and Historical Difference*, Princeton University Press, Princeton, 2000, p. 35.

40 Adam Phillips, *On Flirtation*, Faber & Faber, London, 1994, p. 73.

41 Katie Holmes, *Spaces in Her Day: Australian Women's Diaries 1920s–1930s*, Allen & Unwin, Sydney, pp. xvii–xviii.

42 Baumann, *Modernity and Ambivalence*, p. 4.

43 Kenneth Henderson, 'Emotions: Problems of Management', *Sydney Morning Herald*, 20 July 1935, p. 9.

44 B. S. Jones, Record of Dreams, 1929, entry 'Friday night, December 14th, Burgmann Papers, box 20, file 5.

45 B. S. Jones, Record of Dreams, 1929, entry 'Friday night, 30 November', Burgmann Papers, box 20, file 5.

46 B. S. Jones, Record of Dreams, 1929, entry 'Friday night 14 December', Burgmann Papers, box 20, file 5.

47 B. S. Jones, Record of Dreams, 1929, entry '8 March Friday night', Burgmann Papers, box 20, file 5.

48 McLaren, *Twentieth-Century Sexuality*, p. 112.
49 Porter, *The Interpretation of Dreams*, p. 30.
50 Phillips, *Terrors and Experts*, pp. 64–6.
51 Ruth Bers Shapiro, 'Psychoanalytic Perspectives on Anxiety Dreams in Adults and Children', in Henry Kellerman (ed.), *The Nightmare: Psychological and Biological Foundations*, Columbia University Press, New York, 1987, p. 163.
52 B. S. Jones, Record of Dreams, 1929, entry '16 December', Burgmann Papers, box 20, file 5.
53 B. S. Jones, Record of Dreams, 1929, entry '10 February', Burgmann Papers, box 20, file 5.
54 B. S. Jones, Record of Dreams, 1929, entry 'Sunday night 6 January', Burgmann Papers, box 20, file 5.
55 Reiger, *The Disenchantment of the Home*, pp. 178–9.
56 ibid., p. 188.
57 B. S. Jones, Record of Dreams, 1929, entry '13 February Wednesday night', Burgmann Papers, box 20, file 5.
58 B. S. Jones, Record of Dreams, 1929, entry '9 May', Burgmann Papers, box 20, file 5.
59 Shapiro, 'Psychoanalytic Perspectives', p. 166.
60 Nancy Schnog, 'On Inventing the Psychological', in Pfister and Schnog, *Inventing the Psychological*, p. 8.
61 ibid., p. 3.

3 History, psychoanalysis, modernism

1 Bové, 'Foreword', p. xiii.
2 Bradbury and McFarlane, 'The Name and Nature of Modernism', p. 27.
3 Forrester, *The Seductions of Psychoanalysis*, p. 1.
4 Freud, 'One of the Difficulties of Psycho-analysis', p. 23.
5 Anderson, 'Modernity and Revolution', pp. 104–6.
6 Ryan, *The Vanishing Subject*, p. 2.
7 Jones, 'Editorial', pp. 3–7.
8 Levenson, *A Genealogy of Modernism*, p. 14.
9 Masson, *The Assault on Truth*; Russell, *Women, Madness and Medicine*, pp. 22–4.
10 Forrester, *The Seductions of Psychoanalysis*, p. 79.
11 ibid., p. 81.
12 Eliot, 'Tradition and the Individual Talent'; Pound, 'The Tradition'.
13 Smith, *Modernism's History*, p. 55.
14 Lee, *Virginia Woolf*, pp. 158–9.

4 The inner and outer world of queer life

1 Budd, 'No Sex Please—We're British'.
2 Bersani, *Homos*, p. 19.
3 Butler, 'Moral Sadism and Doubting One's Own Love'.
4 Joan Riviere, 'Womanliness as a Masquerade', *International Journal of Psycho-analysis*, vol. 19, 1929, pp. 193–204.
5 Otero and Escardo, 'Sexuality in the Age of AIDS', pp. 137–8.
6 ibid., p. 138.
7 ibid., p. 139.
8 Abelove, 'Freud, Male Homosexuality and the Americans', p. 381.
9 ibid., p. 382.
10 ibid., p. 389.
11 Frosh, *For and Against Psychoanalysis*, p. 199.
12 Abelove, 'Freud, Male Homosexuality, and the Americans', p. 385.
13 Strozier, *Heinz Kohut*, pp. 265, 341.
14 O'Connor and Ryan, *Wild Desires and Mistaken Identities*, p. 76.
15 ibid., p. 75.

16 ibid., p. 80.
17 ibid., p. 89.
18 Harding, 'Making Sense of Sexuality', p. 8.
19 Isay, *Becoming Gay*, pp. 154–5.
20 Frosh, *For and Against Psychoanalysis*, p. 209.
21 Altman, *Homosexual*, p. 248.
22 Reynolds, *Remaking the Homosexual*.
23 Zaretsky, 'Identity Theory, Identity Politics', p. 200.
24 ibid.
25 Brett, 'The Tasks of Political Biography', in this volume.
26 Reynolds, *Remaking the Homosexual*.
27 Zaretsky, 'Identity Theory, Identity Politics', p. 210.
28 Lane, 'Psychoanalysis and Sexual Identity', p. 164.
29 Chodorow, 'Heterosexuality as a Compromise Formation', p. 269.
30 Giddens, *The Transformation of Intimacy*, p. 179.
31 ibid.
32 Rubin, 'Sexual Traffic', p. 68.
33 Halperin, *Saint Foucault*, p. 91.
34 ibid., p. 97.
35 Rubin, cited in Halperin, *Saint Foucault*, p. 91; O'Carroll, 'Against the Grain', p. 49.
36 O'Carroll, 'Against the Grain', p. 43.
37 ibid.
38 Royston, 'Sexuality and Object Relations', p. 48.
39 <http://www.LeatherViews.com/kinkyinfo/9305.htm>
40 Royston, 'Sexuality and Object Relations', p. 50.

5 Displacing Indigenous Australians

1 Freud, *Totem and Taboo*, p. 53.
2 ibid., p. 54.
3 Deleuze and Guattari, *Anti-Oedipus*, p. 117.
4 Freud, *Beyond the Pleasure Principle*, p. 334.
5 Freud, *Totem and Taboo*, p. 53.
6 Kuklick, *The Savage Within*, p. 280.
7 Pateman, *The Sexual Contract*, p. 1.
8 Barker, *Michel Foucault*, p. 86.
9 ibid., p. 88.
10 ibid., p. 88.
11 ibid., p. 8.
12 Ong, *Orality and Literacy*, p. 12.
13 Kuklick, *The Savage Within*, p. 27.
14 Stocking, *Victorian Anthropology*, p. 158.
15 Cited in ibid., pp. 201–2.
16 Cited in ibid., p. 297.
17 Kuper, *The Invention of Primitive Society*, p. 6.
18 Fison and Howitt, *Kamilaroi and Kurnai*, p. 59.
19 Freud, *Totem and Taboo*, p. 185.
20 ibid., p. 203.
21 ibid., p. 203.
22 Borch-Jacobsen, *The Freudian Subject*, p. 190.
23 Freud, *Totem and Taboo*, p. 217.
24 ibid., p. 124.
25 ibid., p. 62.
26 ibid., p. 70.
27 ibid., p. 104.

[28] Deleuze and Guattari, *Anti-Oedipus*, p. 121.

[29] Freud, *Totem and Taboo*, p. 56n.

[30] ibid., p. 154.

[31] ibid, pp. 70, 189.

[32] ibid., p. 189.

[33] ibid., p. 84.

[34] Freud, *Moses and Monotheism*, p. 283.

[35] Freud, *Civilization and its Discontents*, p. 316.

[36] Freud, 'The Dissection of the Psychical Personality', p. 504.

[37] Freud, *Civilization and its Discontents*, pp. 293–4.

[38] Freud, 'Thoughts for the Times on War and Death', p. 69.

[39] ibid., p. 68.

6 The tasks of political biography

[1] This is a slightly revised version of an essay first published in Judith Brett (ed) *Political Lives*, Allen & Unwin, Sydney, 1997.

[2] Edel, *Writing Lives*, p. 145.

[3] Erikson, 'On "Psycho-Historical Evidence"', in *Life History and the Historical Moment*, p. 158.

[4] Morgan, 'Writing Political Biography', p. 33.

[5] Lasswell, *Psychopathology and Politics*, pp. 76–7; for discussion of Lasswell's theory of the political type, see Davies, *Skills, Outlooks and Passions*, pp. 5–7, 24–50.

[6] Michael Kirby, 'A Reformer's View of Constitutional Monarchy', speech to launch South Australian Branch of Australians for a Constitutional Monarchy, 16 November 1993, p. 2, author's collection.

[7] See discussion of this in Walter, *The Leader*, ch. 1; and I. Donaldson, P. Read and J. Walter (eds), *Shaping Lives: Reflections on Biography*, The Humanities Research Centre, ANU, Canberra, 2002, p. 277.

[8] Horney, *Neurosis and Human Growth*; Tucker, 'A Stalin Biographer's Memoir'.

[9] Kohut, *The Analysis of the Self*, pp. 25–7.

[10] Kohut, 'The Bipolar Self', in *The Restoration of the Self*.

[11] See Brett, *Robert Menzies' Forgotten People*.

[12] Little, 'The Uses of Childhood', pp. 28–32.

[13] Mitchell, *The Selected Melanie Klein*, p. 27.

[14] ibid., p. 29.

[15] Holmes, 'Biographer's Footsteps', p. 2.

[16] Edel, 'The Biographer and Psychoanalysis', pp. 462–3.

7 Reading the Victorian family

[1] Stefan Zweig, *Joseph Fouché: The Portrait of a Politician*, [1930], trans. Eden Paul and Cedar Paul, Guild Books, London 1948, pp. 9, 223–4.

[2] Stefan Zweig, *The World of Yesterday*, [1943], Cassell, London, 1953, pp. 419–24.

[3] John Rickard, *Class and Politics: New South Wales, Victoria and the Early Commonwealth 1890–1910*, ANU Press, Canberra, 1976.

[4] Frank Manuel: in biography most notably the author of *A Portrait of Isaac Newton*, Belknap Press of Harvard University Press, Cambridge, 1986. Saul Friedlander: author of, for example, *Fantasy and Reality in History*, Oxford University Press, New York, 1995.

[5] See, for example, Peter Loewenberg, *Decoding the Past: The Psychohistorical Approach*, Knopf, New York, 1983.

[6] Rickard, *H. B. Higgins*, p. 8.

[7] As suggested by Judith Brett at the seminar of contributors, University of Melbourne, 8 June 2001.

[8] Rickard, *H. B. Higgins*, pp. 11–12.

[9] ibid., p. 12.

[10] These are now further supplemented by the Jessie (Deakin) Clarke Papers held in the State Library of Victoria. The Papers of Alfred and Catherine Deakin, as well as those of Herbert and Ivy Brookes, Deakin's son-in-law and daughter, are in the National Library of Australia.

[11] La Nauze, *Alfred Deakin*, vol. 1, pp. 78–9.

[12] Cited in Rickard, *A Family Romance*, p. 4.

[13] *A New Pilgrim's Progress*, W. H. Terry, Melbourne, 1877. The copy deposited in the State Library of Victoria has long since disappeared, but there is a copy in the Baillieu Library, University of Melbourne.

[14] La Nauze, *Alfred Deakin*, vol. 1, pp. 60–1.

[15] Rickard, *A Family Romance*, p. 43.

[16] Rickard, *H. B. Higgins*, p. 16.

[17] ibid., p. 26.

[18] John Rickard, '"Poor James": An Incident in Irish/Australian History', *Victorian Historical Journal*, 49, no. 4, November 1978, p. 215.

[19] Cited in Rickard, *H. B. Higgins*, p. 185.

[20] Rickard, *A Family Romance*, p. 11.

[21] La Nauze, *Alfred Deakin*, vol. 1, p. 78.

[22] Rickard, *A Family Romance*, pp. 53–4.

[23] H. B. Higgins, *A New Province for Law and Order*, Constable & Co., London, 1922.

[24] Rickard, *H. B. Higgins*, p. 263.

[25] Walter Murdoch, *Alfred Deakin: A Sketch*, Constable & Co., London, 1923.

[26] Peter Gay, *The Bourgeois Experience, Victoria to Freud*, vol. 2, *The Tender Passion*, Oxford University Press, New York, 1986, p. 422.

8 'I knew I would be lonely for them always'

[1] Donald Thomson to William Onus, 11 January 1947, DFT Papers.

[2] *Donald Thomson in Arnhem Land*, p. 107.

[3] Peterson, 'Donald Thomson', pp. vii–viii, 1; Cowlishaw, 'Helping Anthropologists', pp. 12–14.

[4] Henry Reynolds, *This Whispering in Our Hearts*, Allen & Unwin, Sydney, 1998, p. xiv.

[5] Gay, *Freud for Historians*, p. 156. There are few historical sources regarding Thomson's childhood but the voluminous archive for his adult years—and in particular private letters by, to and about Thomson, his reports for government and his articles for newspapers—enable one to undertake a psychoanalytical study. I am indebted to Dorita Thomson for granting me access to her late husband's personal papers, and discussing aspects of his work with me.

[6] Donald Thomson, 'Bird Life in Sherbrooke Gully', *The Scotch Collegian*, vol. XVII, no. 2, 1920, pp. 138, 141.

[7] Donald Thomson, 'A Plea for a Vanishing Race', *Herald*, 22 March 1930; notes and other data relating to photographs, [1933], DT Papers held by Dorita Thomson; Thomson, 'An Arnhem Land Adventure', *Sydney Mail*, 29 December 1937; Thomson, 'Three Years in Arnhem Land, II', *Times*, 6 July 1938. Thomson was an exceptionally fine photographer and this primitivism is evident in many of his images; for examples of these, see Bill Gammage and Peter Spearritt (eds), *Australians 1938*, Fairfax, Syme & Weldon, Sydney, 1987, pp. 66–77.

[8] Inga Clendinnen, *Tiger's Eye*, Text, Melbourne, 2000, p. 209. (She was referring to George Augustus Robinson's relationships with Aborigines).

[9] Thomson to A. R. Radcliffe Brown, 9 April 1929, ANRC Papers, NLA, MS 482/59/847A; Thomson, 'First White Men to Visit Cape York Blacks', *Herald*, 8 June 1929; Thomson, 'A Plea for a Vanishing Race', *Herald*, 22 March 1930; Thomson, 'The Hero Cult, Initiation and Totemism on Cape York', *Journal of the Royal Anthropological Institute*, vol. 63, 1933, pp. 456–7, 459, 471–2; Thomson letter, February 1937, cited in Peterson, 'Donald Thomson', p. 15; Thomson to Fred Goerke, 14 December 1957, DT Papers.

[10] Thomson, notes and other data relating to photographs and Gladys Thomson, Diary, 15–20 December 1932, DT Papers; Peterson, 'Donald Thomson', p. 6; Stuart Macintyre, 'War and

Peace: A History of the College Initiation', in Macintyre (ed.), *Ormond College: Centenary Essays*, Melbourne University Press, Melbourne, 1984, p. 85.

[11] Donald Thomson, draft preface for book by T. T. Webb, 20 April 1934, DT Papers; *Herald*, 14 February 1934; 'My Three Years in the Old Stone Age', *Herald*, 18 August 1934.

[12] Thomson to Charles Duguid, 27 December 1946, Charles Duguid Papers, NLA, MS 5068/1/1; Thomson to Tom Wright, 2 May 1947, Tom and Mary Wright Papers, Noel Butlin Archives Centre, Australian National University, Z267/8; Donald Thomson, 'Wanted—Simple Justice for the Aborigine', *Herald*, 10 April 1950.

[13] There is a considerable body of historical evidence, much of it left by those who regarded Thomson highly and/or loved and respected him, that attests to the fact that he was a troubled man. He was variously described as being 'a nervous excitable individual' and 'a young man with genius, and some of the faults of genius', and as someone who had 'a sensitive nature' and a 'difficult temperament' (Minutes of ANRC Executive Meeting, 27 June 1929; T. G. B. Osborn to Alex J. Gibson, 5 June 1929; David Orme Masson to Osborn, 2 July 1929; Frederick Wood Jones to George Julius, 6 June 1934, ANRC Papers, NLA, MS 482/59/846A, 847A and 847B).

[14] Thomson, 'My Three Years in the Old Stone Age', *Herald*, 18 August 1934.

[15] We know from other incidents in his life that Thomson found situations of this kind intolerable. In 1929 he angrily resigned a research grant when Radcliffe Brown asserted the ANRC's right of ownership over negatives of photographs he had taken the previous year, apparently regarding this as 'an outrageous demand'. One member of the ANRC sympathetic to Thomson astutely observed that the photographs were 'in a peculiar way personal possessions' for him and noted that, however 'absurd', Thomson thought the ANRC was 'attempt[ing] to wrest them from him'; another ally remarked that he had 'lost his head when faced with [a] demand which he thought unfair (Minutes of ANRC Executive Meeting, 27 June 1929; Osborn to Gibson, 5 June 1929, ANRC Papers, NLA MS 482/59/846A and 847B).

[16] Thomson, notes and other data relating to photographs, DT Papers.

[17] Data relating to photographs, DT Papers; Thomson to Duguid, 27 December 1946.

[18] Thomson, General Report of Preliminary Expedition to Arnhem Land, Northern Territory of Australia, 1935–36, p. 35, DFT Papers; Thomson, Recommendations of Policy in Native Affairs in the Northern Territory of Australia, p. 4; Thomson, *Report on Expedition to Arnhem Land*, pp. 10, 14.

[19] Many years later Thomson confessed to Duguid he 'had the Aurukun and MacKenzie business very much on [his] mind' when he took up the position he sought. At the same time, the plight of the Aurukun Aborigines was displaced, at least temporarily, in his mind. In later years he felt guilty for not taking up their cause, trying to excuse his inaction by saying he 'was young then ... had little personal prestige, and ... would of course have been hailed down as a fanatic' (Thomson to Duguid, 15 November 1960, Duguid Papers, NLA, MS 5068/1/2).

[20] J. H. MacFarland to J. A. Perkins, 18 December 1933, NAA, CRS A659, 1939/1/5250.

[21] Thomson to Perkins, 18 July 1934, NAA, CRS A659, 1939/1/5250; *Courier Mail*, 22 March 1935; Thomson, Diary, 27 May 1935, DT Papers.

[22] Thomson, 'Among the Black Killers of Caledon Bay', *Herald*, 1 February 1936; *Herald*, 7 December 1937; *Sydney Morning Herald*, 8 December 1937.

[23] Thomson, 'What Should We Do for the Blacks', *Sun*, 13 January 1940; Thomson, 'Rights of Aborigines', *Herald*, 21 November 1944; Thomson to Robert Menzies, 10 September 1946 and 17 March 1950, DT Papers; Thomson, 'Slow Extermination of Our Natives', *Herald*, 30 December 1946; Thomson, 'Aborigines' Rights to Tribal Lands Should be Recognised', *Herald*, 31 December 1946; Thomson, draft of speech at the University of Melbourne, 27 March 1947, DT Papers; Thomson to Vernon Clark, 29 June 1949, DFT Papers.

[24] Thomson, Heads of Proposals for Agenda for a Conference on Native Rights, *c*. May 1947, DFT Papers.

[25] Thomson, 'Half-Castes Need Our Goodwill', *Herald*, 11 January 1945; Thomson to Onus, 11 January 1947, DFT Papers.

[26] Thomson to Brian Fitzpatrick, 12 December 1946, DFT Papers; Thomson, draft of speech at the University of Melbourne, 27 March 1947, DT Papers; Thomson to Clark, 29 June 1949, DFT Papers.

[27] Thomson, 'Aborigines' "New Deal" is a Raw Deal', *Herald*, 3 April 1946; Thomson to Duguid, 27 December 1946, 15 November 1960, 18 March 1961, Charles Duguid Papers, NLA, MSS 5068/1/1 and 2; *Sydney Daily Telegraph*, 4 April 1950; Thomson to Menzies, 17 March 1950, 20 November 1950, DT Papers; Thomson to John Latham, 22 March 1951, NAA, CRS A452/1, 1954/575.

9 Health, hygiene and the phallic body

[1] William M. Reddy, *The Invisible Code: Honor and Sentiment in Postrevolutionary France, 1814–1848*, University of California Press, Berkeley, 1997, p. 4.

[2] Peter Novick, *That Noble Dream: The 'Objectivity Question' and the American Historical Profession*, Cambridge University Press, Cambridge, 1988, pp. 557–62.

[3] Bryan Turner, *Regulating Bodies: Essays in Medical Sociology*, Routledge, London, 1992, p. 57.

[4] Eric L. Santner, 'My Own Private Germany: Daniel Paul Schreber's Secret History of Modernity,' in Brian Cheyette and Laura Marcus (eds.), *Modernity, Culture, and 'the Jew'*, Polity Press, Cambridge, 1998, p. 40.

[5] Diana Fuss, 'Inside/out', in Diana Fuss (ed.), *Inside/out: Lesbian Theories, Gay Theories*, Routledge, London, 1991, p. 3.

[6] Alan Petersen and Deborah Lupton, *The New Public Health: Health and Self in the Age of Risk*, Allen & Unwin, Sydney, 1996, pp. 61–88.

[7] Foucault, *The History of Sexuality*, vol. 1, Vintage, New York, 1978, p. 152.

[8] Freud, *The Ego and the Id*, Norton, p. 16.

[9] Judith Butler, *Bodies That Matter: On the Discursive Limits of 'Sex'*, Routledge, London, 1993, p. 3; Weiss, *Body Images*, p. 96.

[10] Grosz, *Volatile Bodies*, p. 203.

[11] ibid., p. 58.

[12] The best work on the 'phallic' male body remains Theweleit, *Male Fantasies*.

[13] Bakhtin, *Rabelais and his World*, pp. 317, 26.

[14] Stallybrass and White, *The Politics and Poetics of Transgression*, pp. 144–5.

[15] ibid., p. 29.

[16] Elias, *The Civilizing Process*.

[17] Amiel, *Journal Intime*, vol. VII, 31 March 1870, p. 1359. All translations from this work are my own.

[18] Amiel, *Journal Intime*, vol. IV, April 1861, p. 136.

[19] Amiel, *Journal Intime*, vol. V, 23 August 1863, p. 131; *Journal Intime*, vol. VIII, 22 May 1870, p. 70.

[20] Amiel, *Journal Intime*, vol. II, 1 November 1852, p. 298.

[21] Amiel, *Journal Intime*, vol. VI, 18 April 1866, p. 344.

[22] Amiel, *Journal Intime*, vol. VI, 24 May 1867, p. 908.

[23] John M. Hoberman, 'Otto Weininger and the Critique of Jewish Masculinity', in Nancy A. Harrowitz and Barbara Hyams (eds), *Jews and Gender: Responses to Otto Weininger*, Temple University Press, Philadelphia, 1995, p. 145; Michael Nerlich, *Ideology of Adventure: Studies in Modern Consciousness, 1100–1750*, trans. Ruth Crowley, University of Minnesota Press, Minneapolis, 1987.

[24] Amiel, *Journal Intime*, vol. VII, 19 June 1869, p. 831.

[25] Amiel, *Journal Intime*, vol. VII, 31 March 1870, p. 1359.

[26] Amiel, *Journal Intime*, vol. IX, 10 June 1874, p. 1236.

[27] Amiel, *Journal Intime*, vol. II, 30 April 1855, p. 1055.

[28] Amiel, *Journal Intime*, vol. IX, 9 July 1872, p. 339.

[29] Amiel, *Journal Intime*, vol. VII, 21 September 1868, p. 396.

[30] Amiel, *Journal Intime*, vol. VII, 13 June 1869, p. 818.

[31] Amiel, *Journal Intime*, vol. VII, 21 September 1868, p. 396.

[32] Amiel, *Journal Intime*, vol. VII, 3 December 1868, p. 514.

33 Amiel, *Journal Intime*, vol. II, 31 October 1852, p. 295.
34 Amiel, *Journal Intime*, vol. IX, 2 June 1872, p. 272.
35 Amiel, *Journal Intime*, vol. VII, 17 September 1868, p. 379.
36 See Vernon Rosario, *The Erotic Imagination: French Histories of Perversity*, Oxford University Press, New York, 1997, pp. 24–5.
37 Amiel, *Journal Intime*, vol. VIII, 18 May 1870, p. 59.
38 Amiel, *Journal Intime*, vol. III, 13 July 1860, p. 1045.
39 Amiel, *Journal Intime*, vol. IV, 17 April 1861, pp. 129, 658.
40 Amiel, *Journal Intime*, vol. V, 6 February 1865, p. 837.
41 Amiel, *Journal Intime*, vol. V, 5 June 1865, pp. 990–1.
42 Amiel, *Journal Intime*, vol. XII, 2 May 1880, p. 419.
43 Amiel, *Journal Intime*, vol. III, 13 March 1860, p. 896.
44 Amiel, *Journal Intime*, vol. IV, 25 February 1861, p. 75.
45 Amiel, *Journal Intime*, vol. IX, 16 May 1872, p. 235.
46 Amiel, *Journal Intime*, vol. VIII, 17 May 1870, p. 56.
47 Weiss, *Body Images*, p. 53.

10 Identity: history, the nation and the self

1 Likierman, *Melanie Klein*, pp. 89, 112–14.
2 Paul Ricoeur, 'Myth as the Bearer of Possible Worlds', cited in Richard Kearney, *Postnationalist Ireland: Politics, Culture, Philosophy*, Routledge, London, 1997, p. 225, n. 35.
3 Dixson, *The Real Matilda*; Dixson, *The Imaginary Australian*.
4 Lawrence J. Friedman, *Identity's Architect. A Biography of Erik H. Erikson*, Scribner, New York, 1999, pp. 49, 492, n. 52.
5 For the defining role of relational and moral concerns in the British object-relations tradition, see Joanne Brown and Barry Richards, 'The Humanist Freud', in Anthony Elliott (ed.), *Freud 2000*, Melbourne University Press, Melbourne, 1998, pp. 235–61. For Winnicott, see Dixson, *The Imaginary Australian*, pp. 4–5, 20–1 and *passim*.
6 Erikson, *Childhood and Society*, ch. 7, 'Eight Ages of Man', pp. 239–66.
7 Louis Hartz, *The Founding of New Societies: Studies in the History of the United States, Latin America, South Africa, Canada, and Australia*, Harcourt, Brace & World, New York, 1964.
8 W. K. Hancock, *Australia*, Ernest Benn, London, 1945, p. 36.
9 On respectability, see Miriam Dixson, 'Gender, Class and the Women's Movements in Australia, 1890, 1980', in Norma Grieve and Ailsa Burns (eds), *Australian Women: New Feminist Perspectives*, Oxford University Press, Melbourne, 1986, pp. 18–21.
10 See Dixson, *The Imaginary Australian*, pp. 50–6.
11 See Robert Dessaix's experience in making a Radio National program on Australian public intellectuals: 'Hail the tall poppy', *Sydney Morning Herald*, 10 May 1997.
12 Peter Cotton, 'Manning Clark on Life, Politics and the Quest for Grace', *The National Graduate*, vol. 2, no. 1, 1991, pp. 7–8; also cited in Miriam Dixson, 'Clark and National Identity', in Carl Bridge (ed.), *Manning Clark: Essays on his Place in History*, Melbourne University Press, Melbourne, 1994, p. 194.
13 Dorothy Dinnerstein, *The Mermaid and The Minotaur: Sexual Arrangements and Human Malaise*, Harper and Row, New York, 1976.
14 Melanie Klein, 'The Development of a Child', [1921], in *Love, Guilt and Reparation*, The Hogarth Press, London, 1975, p. 52.
15 Melanie Klein, 'A Contribution to the Psychogenesis of Manic-depressive States', [1935], in *Love, Guilt and Reparation*, p. 286.
16 Anthony Elliott, 'Philosopher of Passion', *Australian*, 1 April 1998.
17 The work of Castoriadis most directly relevant to this chapter is *The Imaginary Institution of Society*.
18 For their generous help on Castoriadis, my grateful thanks to Dr. Sue Rechter, Department of Sociology, Australian Catholic University, and to Professor Johann Arnason, Department of Sociology and Anthropology, La Trobe University, Victoria.

[19] Dixson, *The Imaginary Australian*, pp. 19–20.

[20] Castoriadis, *The Imaginary Institution of Society*, pp. 128–30.

11 Psychoanalytic theory and sources of national attachment

[1] The term is used by Kristeva in *Nations without Nationalism*, trans. Leon S. Roudiez, Columbia University Press, New York, 1993.

[2] Anderson, *Imagined Communities*.

[3] See Castoriadis, *World in Fragments*, ch. 1.

[4] Anthony Elliott, *Subject to Ourselves: Social Theory, Psychoanalysis and Postmodernism*, Polity Press, Cambridge, 1996, pp. 8–38.

[5] Dixson, *The Imaginary Australian*, p. 50.

[6] Kohut, *The Analysis of the Self*.

[7] Dixson, *The Imaginary Australian*, p. 55.

[8] Lefebvre, *The Production of Space*.

12 Contemporary fantasies of ancient hatred

[1] Sadkovich, *The U.S. Media and Yugoslavia*, p. 125.

[2] Freud, *Thoughts for the Times on War and Death*, p. 130.

[3] Cash, *Identity, Ideology and Conflict*, p. 37.

[4] The notion of ideological fantasy is taken from the work of Slavoj Zizek.

[5] Laclau 'The Death and Resurrection of the Theory of Ideology', p. 304.

[6] Zizek, *The Plague of Fantasies*, p. 4 (italicised in original).

[7] White House Press Secretary, Michael McCurry, *White House Press Briefing*, 15 August 1997 (Reuters).

[8] Michel Feher, *Powerless by Design*, p. 40.

[9] ibid., p. 39.

[10] 'CNN Interview with President of Serbia Slobodan Milosevic', 22 December 1994, <http://www.yugoslavia.com/Bulletin/95/95jan/95jan4.htm> (accessed 28 February 1999).

[11] ibid.

[12] Thompson, *Forging War*, p. 51.

[13] ICTY Indictment of Radovan Karadzic and Ratko Mladic, <http://www.un.org/icty/indictment/english/karii950724e.htm> (accessed on 6 August 2001).

[14] ICTY Indictment of Biljana Plavsic <http://www.un.org/icty/english/pla-ii00047e.htm> (accessed on 6 August 2001).

[15] 'Declaration of the Assembly of Citizens of Serbian Nationality and of Serb Ethnic Origin, and Appeal to the Citizens and Peoples of the Republic of Bosnia and Herzegovina to summon the Convention of Confidence', 27 March 1994, in Snezana Trifunovska (ed.), *Yugoslavia Through Documents: From its Creation to its Dissolution*, Martinus Nijhoff Publishers, Dordrech, Boston, p. 121.

[16] David Owen, 'Dramatis Personae', in *Balkan Odyssey*, Indigo, London, 1996.

[17] Feher, *Powerless by Design*, p. 48.

[18] Owen, *Balkan Odyssey*, p. 52.

[19] Ramet, *Balkan Babel*, p. 248.

[20] Feher, *Powerless by Design*, p. 81.

[21] Campbell, *National Deconstruction*, p. 128.

[22] ibid.

[23] ibid., p. 140.

[24] Etiene Balibar, 'Is there a Neo-Racism?' in Etiene Balibar and Immanuel Wallerstein (eds), *Race, Nation, Class: Ambiguous Identities*, Verso, London, 1991, p. 21.

[25] ibid., p. 21.

[26] ibid., p. 22.

[27] ibid., p. 25.

28 Tone R. Bringa, 'National Categories, National Identification and Identity Formation in "Multi-national" Bosnia', *Anthropology of East Europe Review*, vol. 11, nos 1–2 Autumn 1993, p. 2.
29 Quoted in Campbell, *National Deconstruction*, p. 144.
30 Kemal Kurspahic quoted in Campbell, *National Deconstruction*, p. 144.
31 Noel Malcolm, 'The Bosnian blood on Douglas Hurd's hands: Our policy in the Balkans has been a disaster', *Sunday Telegraph London*, 13 February 1994.
32 Feher, *Powerless by Design*, p. 123.

13 'Impossible history'

1 Civilian internees' names used throughout this chapter are pseudonyms. The correspondence cited is on public record at the National Archives of Australia (NAA), located at the file references cited hereafter.
2 Mrs G. K. to Secretary, CITF, 25 August 1957, NAA, CA 2434 CITF, series B510, Application forms for grants and associated documents [CITF] no. 334.
3 For brief references see Hank Nelson, *P.O.W. Prisoners of War: Australians Under Nippon*, ABC Enterprises, Sydney, 1985, p. 77; and Patsy Adam-Smith, *Prisoners of War: From Gallipoli to Korea*, Viking, Melbourne, 1992.
4 'Statement "A": Analysis of the Total Number of Australian Civilian Internees by Location of Internment', in CITF, Final Report: Covering the Operations of the Trust 1952–1962, 29 October 1962, typescript, NAA, series B512/1, box 1, see Michael P. Tracey (ed.), *Australian Prisoners of War*, special issue of *Australian Defence Force Journal*, Department of Defence, Canberra, 1999, p. 102.
5 Cathy Caruth, 'Trauma and Experience: Introduction', in Caruth, *Trauma*, p. 4.
6 Dominick LaCapra, 'Trauma, Absence, Loss', *Critical Enquiry*, vol. 25, issue 4, Summer 1999, online version, Expanded Academic ASAP, paragraphs 33, 34, 35.
7 Caruth, 'Trauma and Experience', in Caruth, *Trauma*, pp. 4–5.
8 Eve ten Brummelaar, *You Can't Eat Grass*, Image DTP and Printing, Sydney, 1996, p. 80.
9 Caruth, 'Trauma and Experience', in Caruth, *Trauma*, p. 5.
10 Brummelaar, *You Can't Eat Grass*, p. 81.
11 Dori Laub, 'Truth and Testimony: The Process and the Struggle' in Caruth, *Trauma*, p. 64.
12 Bessel A. Van der Kolk and Onno Van der Hart, 'The Intrusive Past: The Flexibility of Memory and the Engraving of Trauma', in Caruth, *Trauma*, p. 176.
13 press release, [no number], by Acting Prime Minister [Fadden], 8 December 1952, 'Civilian Internees Trust Fund', NAA, series B512, 52/68. The fund was established under Section 13 F (3) of the *Trading with the Enemy Act 1939–1957*.
14 CITF, Final Report: Covering the Operations of the Trust 1952–1962, 29 October 1962, typescript, NAA, series B512/1, box 1.
15 The Civilian Internees Trust Fund Application for a Grant, NAA, series B512/1.
16 M. M. to CITF, 15 January 1953, NAA, series B510, no. 258.
17 Mrs E. R. to Professor F. A. Bland, MHR, 21 December 1853, NAA, series B510, no. 286.
18 NAA, series B510, no. 281.
19 Mrs R. T. to CITF, 11 August 1953, NAA, series B510, no. 296.
20 NAA, series B510, no. 255.
21 NAA, series B510, no. 196.
22 E. R. to Professor Bland, MHR, 21 December 1953, NAA, series B510, no. 286.
23 C. J. to CITF, 9 February 1953, NAA, series B510, no. 268.
24 NAA, series B510, no. 184.
25 NAA, series B510, no. 256.
26 NAA, series B510, no. 229.
27 NAA, series B510, no. 329.
28 Dr W. L. Kirkwood, Statement, 24 January 1953, NAA, series B510, no. 290.
29 A. I. to CITF, 17 February 1953, NAA, series B510, no. 245.
30 NAA, series B510.

³¹ M. W-L. to CITF, 10 June 1953, NAA, series B510, no. 181.

³² Mrs M. M. to Secretary, CITF, 15 January 1953, NAA, series B510, no. 258.

³³ NAA, series B13/0, 1934/7225.

³⁴ SLV, La Trobe Picture Collection, Argus Collection, box 27A, H98 103/3212; H98/103/3224.

³⁵ F. M. to Treasurer, 12 May 1945, NAA, series A1379/1, EPJ1107.

³⁶ NAA, series A13791, EPJ1108.

³⁷ Draft of a Letter to Mrs M. contained in Prime Minister's Department to Mr J. Kelly, Private Secretary to the Treasurer, 12 Dec 1952, NAA, series B510, no. 258.

³⁸ NAA, series A13791, EPJ1108.

³⁹ Joy Damousi, *Living With the Aftermath: Trauma, Nostalgia and Grief in Post-war Australia*, Cambridge University Press, Cambridge, UK, 2001, p. 3.

14 Let's stop enjoying the Holocaust

¹ Lily Brett, cited in Simon Mann, 'Breaking the Wall of Silence', *Age*, Extra, 7 April 2001, p. 8.

² Lily Brett, 'Surviving Germany', *Age*, Extra, 10 July 1999, pp. 4, 6.

³ On Jews redeeming Germans of their past, see Susanne Klingenstein, 'Visits to Germany in Recent Jewish-American Writing', *Contemporary Literature*, vol. 34, no. 3, 1993, pp. 538–70.

⁴ Sigmund Freud, 'The "Uncanny"' (1919), in *Standard Edition XVII*, ed. and trans. James Strachey, The Hogarth Press, London, 1955. *Heimisch* comes from the same root as *heimlich* and in this context means homelike, domestic, with the emphasis on comfortableness and snugness; *heimlich* incorporates these meanings but has a number of added meanings, such as secretive, concealed, private and underhand. Freud's lengthy teasing out of all the denotations and connotations of *unheimlich* in his essay 'The "Uncanny"' exposes the familia(l)r core of what is most strange and frightening, and *vice versa*.

⁵ Cathy Caruth, 'Unclaimed Experience: Trauma and the Possibility of History', *Yale French Studies*, no. 79, 1991, pp. 181–92.

⁶ Jacques Lacan, Seminar on Anxiety 1962–1963, The Seminar of Jacques Lacan, Book X, trans. Cormac Gallagher from unedited Franch typescripts, session of 28 Nov. 1962, p. 5. See also Jacques Lacan, 'The Function and Field of Speech and Language in Psychoanalysis', in *Ecrits: A Selection*, trans. Alan Sheridan, Tavistock/Routledge, London, 1977, pp. 51–2; Jacques-Alain Miller, 'Suture (Elements of the Logic of the Signifier)', *Screen*, vol. 18, no. 4, 1977/8, pp. 24–34.

⁷ For the way these terms, 'real' and '*jouissance*', are used in Lacanian psychoanalysis, see Lacan, *The Four Fundamental Concepts of Psycho-Analysis*; Lacan, *On Feminine Sexuality*.

⁸ Lacan, *The Ethics of Psychoanalysis*.

⁹ Jaanus, '"A Civilisation of Hatred"', p. 344.

¹⁰ Fein, *April Fool*.

¹¹ For a concise account of this episode in Australian history and of its continuing effects, see Suzanne D. Rutland, *Edge of the Diaspora: Two Centuries of Jewish Settlement in Australia*, 2nd rev. ed., Brandl & Schlesinger, Sydney, 1997, pp. 245–51, 390–1, 399–400. A fuller discussion is provided in Mark Aarons, *Sanctuary: Nazi Fugitives in Australia*, William Heinemann Australia, Melbourne, 1989.

¹² Sigmund Freud, 'On Narcissism: An Introduction', [1914], in *Standard Edition XIV*, ed. and trans. James Strachey, The Hogarth Press, London, 1957; and Sigmund Freud, *Group Psychology and the Analysis of the Ego*, [1921], *Standard Edition XVIII*, ed. and trans. James Strachey, The Hogarth Press, London, 1955, ch. 8.

¹³ Freud, *The Ego and the Id*, in *Standard Edition XIX*, p. 50, n. 1.

¹⁴ Yvonne Fein, talk to Descendants of the Shoah (DOSINC), 1992, audiotape held by Makor Library.

¹⁵ David Gerber, 'Of Mice and Men: Cartoons, Metaphors, and Children of Holocaust Survivors in Recent Jewish Experience: A Review Essay', *American Jewish History*, vol. 77, 1987, pp. 159–75.

16 Jacqueline Rose, *The Haunting of Sylvia Plath*, Virago, London, 1991, pp. 205–38; Klein and Kogan, 'Identification Processes and Denial in the Shadow of Nazism'. See also Marion M. Oliner, 'Hysterical Features Among Children of Survivors' and Maria V. Bergmann, 'Thoughts on Superego Pathology of Survivors and Their Children', both in Martin S. Bergmann and Milton E. Jucovy (eds), *Generations of the Holocaust*, Columbia University Press, New York, pp. 267–86 and 287–309; Dinora Pines, 'The Impact of the Holocaust on the Second Generation', in *A Woman's Unconscious Use of Her Body*, Yale University Press, New Haven, Conn., 1994, pp. 205–25.

17 Interview with Yvonne Fein at Melbourne Jewish Holocaust Museum and Research Centre, February 1999, videotape held by author and Museum.

18 Fein, talk to DOSINC, 1992.

19 Jaanus, '"A Civilisation of Hatred"', p. 346.

20 Fein, talk to DOSINC, 1996, audiotape held by Makor Library.

21 Interview with Fein, 1999; Fein, talk to DOSINC, 1992.

22 Fein, *April Fool*, p. 191.

23 Interview with Fein, 1999.

24 Fein, 'Disclaimer', *April Fool*.

25 The names that appear in the novel correspond to real family names. Personal communication by author, May 2001.

26 Alana Rosenbaum, 'Writing Out Survivor Guilt', *Australian Jewish News*, 30 March 2001, p. 9.

27 Jacques Lacan, Seminar on Anxiety 1962–1963, The Seminar of Jacques Lacan, Book X, ed. and trans. Cormac Gallagher from unedited French typescripts, session 14 Nov. 1962, p. 10; Vicente Palomera, '"*Das Ding*" and Sublimation', *Analysis*, vol. 6, 1995, pp. 115–19.

28 Fein, *April Fool*, p. 168.

29 ibid., p. 265.

30 ibid., p. 304.

31 ibid., p. 22.

32 Zev Garber and Bruce Zuckerman, 'Why Do We Call the Holocaust "The Holocaust"? An Inquiry into the Psychology of Labels', in Yehuda Bauer et al. (eds), *Remembering for the Future: Working Papers and Addenda*, vol. 2, *The Impact of the Holocaust on the Contemporary World*, Pergamon Press, Oxford, 1989, pp. 1884–6.

33 Fein, *April Fool*, p. 21. This term refers to the German Federal Republic's decision in the 1950s to make financial restitution to the victims of the Nazi regime, for damage to their physical and mental health.

34 ibid., p. 81.

35 ibid., p. 65.

36 ibid., pp. 217–18.

37 ibid., p. 175.

38 ibid., p. 173.

39 ibid., p. 175.

40 ibid., p. 343.

41 Fein, talk to DOSINC, 1992.

42 Klein and Kogan, 'Identification and Denial in the Shadow of Nazism', pp. 48–50.

43 Her testimony makes much of her parents' heroic stories.

44 Fein, *April Fool*, p. 23.

45 ibid., p. 34.

46 ibid., p. 5.

47 ibid., p. 192.

48 ibid., p. 84.

49 ibid., pp. 88–9.

50 My thanks to Silvia Rodríguez for pointing this out. On the fascist aesthetic, see Susan Sontag, 'Fascinating Fascism', [1972], in *Under the Sign of Saturn*, Farrar, Strauss, Giroux, New York, 1980, pp. 73–105.

51 Fein, *April Fool*, p. 341.

52 Sigmund Freud, 'The Economic Problem of Masochism', [1924], in *Standard Edition XIX*, ed. and trans. James Strachey, The Hogarth Press, London, 1961; Sigmund Freud, ' "A Child is Being Beaten". A Contribution to the Study of the Origin of Sexual Perversions', [1919], in *Standard Edition XVII*, ed. and trans. James Strachey, The Hogarth Press, London 1955.

53 Jacques Lacan, The Other Side of Psychoanalysis 1969–1970, The Seminar of Jacques Lacan, Book XVII, unpub. text estab. Jacques-Alain Miller, trans. Russell Grigg, ch. 3, p. 33. See also Freud, *The Ego and The Id*, in *Standard Edition XIX*, ch. 111.

54 Dr Marc Strauss, Lacan Seminar, Australian Centre for Psychoanalysis, Melbourne, April 2001.

55 This question was formulated as such by Dr Marc Strauss.

56 Fein, *April Fool*, pp. 61, 171, 201. 'If love aspires to the unfolding of the being of the other, hate wishes the opposite ... That is what makes hate a career with no limit, just as love is.' Jacques Lacan, *Freud's Papers on Technique 1953–1954*, The Seminar of Jacques Lacan, Book 1, ed. Jacques-Alain Miller, trans. John Forrester, p. 277, cited in Jaanus, ' "A Civilisation of Hatred" ', p. 344.

57 Yvonne Fein, 'Running Writing', *Antipodes: A North American Journal of Australian Literature*, vol. 5, no. 2, December 1991, p. 141.

58 Fein, *April Fool*, p. 138.

59 Joan Copjec, 'The Tomb of Perseverance: On *Antigone*', in *Giving Ground: The Politics of Propinquity*, Verso, New York, 1999, p. 256.

60 ibid., p. 268.

61 Eva Hoffman, *Lost in Translation: Life in a New Language*, Vintage, London, 1998, p. 230.

62 *Australian Jewish News*, 30 March 2001, p. 9.

63 Interview with Fein 1999.

64 Sigmund Freud, 'Instincts and their Vicissitudes', [1905], in *Standard Edition XIV*, ed. and trans. James Strachey, The Hogarth Press, London, 1957, p. 139.

65 Freud, *The Ego and the Id*, in *Standard Edition XIX*, p. 42.

66 Fein, *April Fool*, p. 123.

67 Lacan, *The Ethics of Psychoanalysis*, ch. 11.

68 Andrew Lewis, 'From the Work of Transference to the Transference of Work', *Analysis*, vol. 9, 2000, p. 143.

69 Copjec, 'The Tomb of Perseverance', p. 260.

70 Lacan, *The Ethics of Psychoanalysis*, pp. 72, 112, 125, 141.

71 Esther Faye, 'Story, h/History, Historiality: Memoir as the Writing of Trauma', *Meridian*, vol. 16, no. 2, 1997, pp. 315–39.

72 Fein, *April Fool*, p. 354.

73 ibid., p. 357.

74 ibid., p. 338.

75 ibid., p. 358.

76 Freud, *The Ego and the Id*, in *Standard Edition XIX*, p. 53.

77 Yvonne Fein, 'Orthodox Girls Embrace the Torah', *Australian Jewish News*, 1 June 2001, p. 6.

78 Marianne Hirsch, 'Pictures of a Displaced Girlhood', in *Family Frames: Photography, Narrative and Postmemory*, Harvard University Press, Cambridge, Mass., 1997.

15 Narratives, terminable and interminable

1 Sigmund Freud, 'Recollection, Repetition and Working Through', in *Further Recommendations in the Technique of Psychoanalysis*, p. 158.

2 ibid., p. 159.

3 For example, 'The patient cannot remember the whole of what is repressed in him, and what he cannot remember may be precisely the essential part of it ...' (Sigmund Freud, *Beyond the Pleasure Principle*, p. 288).

4 Freud, 'Analysis Terminable and Interminable', pp. 260–1.

5 ibid., p. 261.

6 See Peter Brooks's discussion of the relation between desire and plot/conclusion within narrative in 'Freud's Masterplot', pp. 280–300.

7 See for example Jacques Derrida's discussion of this in 'Freud and the Scene of Writing', in *Writing and Difference*, p. 211.

8 See Derrida's use of Levi-Strauss's term in 'Structure, Sign and Play', in *Writing and Difference*, p. 285.

9 Atwood, *Alias Grace*, p. 22.

10 ibid., p. 53.

11 ibid., p. 85.

12 Freud, *Beyond the Pleasure Principle*, p. 288.

13 Atwood, *Alias Grace*, p. 103.

14 ibid., p. 133.

15 Margaret Rogerson, 'Reading the Patchworks', p. 6 and *passim*.

16 Emily Dickinson, 'Tell all the Truth but tell it slant—', p. 248.

17 Freud, *Beyond the Pleasure Principle*, p. 307.

18 Atwood, *Alias Grace*, p. 122.

19 ibid., pp. 129, 280.

20 ibid., p. 179.

21 ibid., p. 313.

22 ibid., p. 155.

23 ibid., p. 459.

24 Rogerson, 'Reading the Patchworks', p. 21.

25 Atwood, *Alias Grace*, p. 459.

26 ibid., p. 460.

27 Derrida, *Writing and Difference*, p. 292.

Conclusion: politics, history and the unconscious

1 J. Elster, *The Cement of Society*, p. vii.

2 J. Benjamin, *The Bonds of Love*, pp. 87–8.

3 R. Rorty, 'The Contingency of Selfhood' in *Contingency, Irony and Solidarity*, p. 35.

4 The reference is to William Blake's 'London': 'I wander thro' each charter'd street,/Near where the charter'd Thames does flow/And mark in every face I meet/Marks of weakness, marks of woe.'

5 Philip Larkin, quoted in Rorty, 'The Contingency of Selfhood', in *Contingency, Irony and Solidarity*, p. 23.

6 Dennis Wrong, 'The Oversocialized Conception of Man in Modern Sociology', in *Skeptical Sociology*, Columbia University Press, New York, 1976, pp. 31–46. See a similar discussion of this point in Peter Gay, *Freud for Historians*, ch. 5.

7 Wrong, 'The Oversocialized Conception of Man in Modern Sociology', p. 37.

8 E. Fromm, 'Theory and Method of an Analytic Social Psychology', in Arato and Gebhardt, *The Essential Frankfurt School Reader*, pp. 477–96.

9 Goldhagen, *Hitler's Willing Executioners*, p. 46.

10 ibid., p. 416.

11 H. Dicks, 'Personality Traits and National Socialist Ideology', in DiRenzo, *Personality and Politics*, p. 162.

12 See the discussion in Goldhagen, *Hitler's Willing Executioners*, pp. 444–7, for instance.

13 Adorno, *The Culture Industry*, ch. 5.

14 Althusser, *Lenin and Philosophy*, pp. 127–86.

15 ibid., pp. 154–5.

16 ibid., p. 133.

Bibliography

Abelove, Henry, 'Freud, Male Homosexuality, and the Americans', in H. Abelove et al. (eds), *The Lesbian and Gay Studies Reader*, Routledge, New York, 1995, pp. 381–93.

Adorno, T. W. et al., *The Authoritarian Personality*, Norton, New York, 1969.

Adorno, T. W., *The Culture Industry*, Routledge, London, 1991.

Alexander, Sally, 'Women, Class and Sexual Difference in the 1830s and '40s: Some Reflections on the Writing of a Feminist History', *History Workshop Journal*, vol. 17, 1984, pp. 125–49.

——, *Becoming a Woman And Other Essays in 19th and 20th Century Feminist History*, Virago, London, 1994.

Althusser, L., *Lenin and Philosophy*, Monthly Review Press, New York, 1971.

Altman, Dennis, *Homosexual: Oppression and Liberation*, New York University Press, New York, 1971.

——, *Global Sex*, Allen & Unwin, Sydney, 2001.

Amiel, Henri-Frédéric, *Journal Intime*, vols II–XII, ed. Bernard Gagnebin and Philippe M. Monnier, L'Age d'Homme, Lausanne, 1978–94.

Anderson, Benedict, *Imagined Communities: Reflections on the Origins and Spread of Nationalism*, Verso, London, 1983.

Anderson, Perry, 'Modernity and Revolution', *New Left Review*, no. 144, March–April 1984, pp. 96–113.

Antze, Paul and Lambeck, Michael (eds), *Tense Past: Cultural Essays in Trauma and Memory*, Routledge, London, 1996.

Arato, A. and Gebhardt, E. (eds), *The Essential Frankfurt School Reader*, Urizen Books, New York, 1978.

Archer, Bernice, '"A Low Key Affair": Memories of Civilian Internment in the Far East, 1942–45', in Martin Evans and Ken Lunn (eds), *War and Memory in the Twentieth Century*, Berg, Oxford, 1997.

Attwood, Bain, *Rights for Aborigines*, Allen & Unwin, Sydney, 2003, chapter 5.

——, 'Anthropology, Aboriginality and Aboriginal Rights', in Nicolas Peterson and Bruce Rigsby (eds), *'Tons and Tons of Material': Donald Thomson, the Man and the Scholar*, Australian Academy of the Social Sciences, Canberra, in press.

Atwood, Margaret, *Alias Grace*, Bloomsbury, London, 1996.

Bakhtin, Mikhail, *Rabelais and his World*, trans. Hélène Iswolsky, Indiana University Press, Bloomington, Ind., 1984.

Bal, Mieke, Crewe, Jonathon and Spitzer, Leo (eds), *Acts of Memory: Cultural Recall and the Present*, University Press of New England, Hanover, N.H., 1999.

Barker, Philip, *Michel Foucault: Subversions of the Subject*, Allen & Unwin, Sydney, 1994.

Baumann, Zygmut, *Modernity and Ambivalence*, Polity Press, London, 1991.

Benjamin, J., *The Bonds of Love*, Pantheon Books, New York, 1988.

Bersani, Leo, *Homos*, Harvard University Press, Cambridge, Mass., 1995.

Blackman, Lisa M., 'What Is Doing History? The Use of History to Understand the Constitution of Contemporary Psychological Objects', *Theory & Psychology*, vol. 4, no. 4, 1994, pp. 485–504.

Borch-Jacobsen, Mikkel, *The Freudian Subject*, trans. Catherine Porter, Macmillan, London, 1987.

Bové, Paul, Foreword, 'The Foucault Phenomenon: The Problematics of Style', in Gilles Deleuze, *Foucault*, trans. and ed. Sean Hand, University of Minnesota Press, Minneapolis, Minn., 1988.

Bradbury, Malcolm and McFarlane, James, 'The Name and Nature of Modernism', in Malcolm Bradbury and James McFarlane (eds), *Modernism 1890–1930*, Harvester Press, Atlantic Highlands, N.J., 1978.

Brett, Judith, 'Psychoanalysis in Australia', *Meanjin*, vol. 41, no. 3, September 1982, pp. 339–341.

——, *Robert Menzies' Forgotten People*, Macmillan Australia, Sydney, 1992.

Brooks, Peter, 'Freud's Masterplot', in Shoshana Felman (ed.), *Literature and Psychoanalysis: The Question of Reading, Otherwise*, Johns Hopkins University Press, Baltimore, Md, 1982, pp. 280–300.

Budd, Susan, 'No Sex Please—We're British: Sexuality in English and French Psychoanalysis', in C. Harding (ed.), *Sexuality: Psychoanalytic Perspectives*, Brunner-Routledge, Hove, 2001, pp. 52–68.

Burgmann, Ernest, Papers, National Library of Australia, MS 1998.

Burnham, John C., 'Psychoanalysis and American Medicine, 1894–1918: Medicine, Science, and Culture', in M. Grene (ed.), *Toward a Unity of Knowledge*, Psychological Issues, vol. 6, no. 2, monograph 22, International Universities Press, New York, 1969.

Butler, Judith, 'Moral Sadism and Doubting One's Own Love: Kleinian Reflections on Melancholia', in J. Phillips and L. Stonebridge (eds), *Reading Melanie Klein*, Routledge, London, 1998, pp. 179–89.

Campbell, David, *National Deconstruction: Violence, Identity and Justice in Bosnia*, Minnesota University Press, Minneapolis, 1998.

Caruth, Cathy (ed.), *Trauma: Explorations in Memory*, Johns Hopkins University Press, Baltimore, Md, 1995.

——, *Unclaimed Experience: Trauma, Narrative and History*, Johns Hopkins University Press, Baltimore, Md, 1996.

Casey, Edward, *Getting Back into Place: Towards a Renewed Understanding of the Place-world*, Indiana University Press, Bloomington, Ind., 1993.

Cash, John, *Identity, Ideology and Conflict: the Structuration of Politics in Northern Ireland*, Cambridge University Press, New York, 1996.

Castoriadis, Cornelius, *The Imaginary Institution of Society*, [1975], trans. Kathleen Blamey, Polity Press, Cambridge, 1987.

——, *World in Fragments: Writings on Politics, Society, Psychoanalysis and the Imagination*, ed. and trans. David Ames Curtis, Stanford University Press, Stanford, Calif., 1997.

Certeau, Michel de, *Heterologies: Discourse on the Other*, trans. Brian Massumi, University of Minnesota Press, Minneapolis, Minn., 1986.

Chodorow, Nancy, 'Heterosexuality as a Compromise Formation: Reflections on the Psychoanalytic Theory of Sexual Development', *Psychoanalysis and Contemporary Thought*, vol. 15, 1992, pp. 267–304.

Cowlishaw, Gillian, 'Helping Anthropologists: Cultural Continuity in the Constructions of Aboriginalists', *Canberra Anthropology*, vol. 13, no. 2, 1990, pp. 1–28.

Currie, Anne Catherine, 1845–1908, Farm Diaries 1873–1916, 7 vols, State Library of Victoria, La Trobe Australian Manuscripts Collection, MS 10886 MSB623.

Curthoys, Ann, 'Eugenics, Feminism, and Birth Control: The Case of Marion Piddington', *Hecate*, vol. 15, no.1, 1989, pp. 73–89.

Cushman, Philip, *Constructing the Self, Constructing America: A Cultural History of Psychotherapy*, Addison-Wesley, Boston, 1995.

Darwin, Charles, *The Origin of Species*, [1859], ed. Gillian Beer, Oxford University Press, Oxford, 1996.

——, *The Descent of Man and Selection in Relation to Sex*, John Murray, London, 1901.

Davidoff, Leonore, 'Class and Gender in Victorian England: The Case of Hannah Cullwick and AJ Munby', in *Worlds Between: Historical Perspectives on Gender and Class*, Polity Press, Cambridge, 1995, pp. 103–50.

——, 'Where the Stranger Begins: The Questions of Siblings in Historical Analysis', in *Worlds Between: Historical Perspectives on Gender and Class*, Polity Press, Cambridge, 1995, pp. 206–26.

Davies, A. F., *Skills, Outlooks and Passions*, Cambridge University Press, Cambridge, 1981.

Deleuze, Gilles and Guattari, Felix, *Anti-Oedipus: Capitalism and Schizophrenia*, trans. Robert Hurley, Mark Seem and Helen R. Lane, University of Minnesota Press, Minneapolis, Minn., 1983.

Derrida, Jacques, *Writing and Difference*, University of Chicago Press, Chicago, 1978.

Dickinson, Emily, 'Tell all the Truth but tell it slant—', in *Final Harvest: Emily Dickinson's Poems*, ed. Thomas H. Johnson, Little Brown, Boston, 1961, pp. 248–9.

DiRenzo, G. J., *Personality and Politics*, Anchor Books, New York, 1974.

Dixson, Miriam, *The Imaginary Australian: Anglo-Celts and Identity—1788 to the Present*, University of New South Wales Press, Sydney 1999.

——, *The Real Matilda: Women and Identity in Australia, 1788 to the Present*, 4th edn, University of New South Wales Press, Sydney, 1999.

During, Simon, 'Rousseau's Patrimony: Primitivism, Romance and Becoming Other', in F. Barker, P. Hulme and M. Iverson (eds), *Colonial Discourse/Postcolonial Theory*, Manchester University Press, Manchester, 1994, pp. 47–71.

Edel, Leon, 'The Biographer and Psychoanalysis', *International Journal of Psychoanalysis*, vol. 42, 1961, pp. 458–66.

——, *Writing Lives: Principia Biographica*, W. W. Norton, New York, 1984.

Elias, Norbert, *The Civilizing Process*, Blackwell, London, 1994.

Eliot, T. S., 'Tradition and the Individual Talent', in T. S. Eliot, *The Sacred Wood: Essays on Poetry and Criticism*, [1920], Methuen, London, 1934.

Elliott, Anthony, *Psychoanalytic Theory: An Introduction*, Blackwell, Oxford, 1994.

Elster, J., *The Cement of Society*, Cambridge University Press, Cambridge, UK, 1989.

Erikson, E., *Childhood and Society*, W. W. Norton, New York, 1963.

——, *Childhood and Society*, Penguin, Harmondsworth, 1965.

——, *Life History and the Historical Moment*, W. W. Norton, New York, 1975.

Fabian, Johannes, *Time and the Other: How Anthropology Makes its Object*, Columbia University Press, New York, 1983.

Feher, Michel, *Powerless by Design: The Age of the International Community*, Duke University Press, Durham, Calif., 2000.

Fein, Yvonne, *April Fool: An April Taub Investigation*, Hodder, Sydney, 2001.

Felman, Shoshana and Laub, Dori (eds), *Testimony: Crises of Witnessing in Literature, Psychoanalysis and History*, Routledge, New York, 1992.

Figlio, Karl, 'Historical Imagination/Psychoanalytic Imagination', *History Workshop Journal*, no. 45, 1998, pp. 199–221.

Fison, Lorimer and Howitt, Alfred William, *Kamilaroi and Kurnai: Group Marriage and Relationship, and Marriage by Elopement, Drawn Chiefly from the Usage of the Australian Aborigines, also the Kurnai Tribe: Their Customs in Peace and War*, George Robertson, Melbourne, 1880.

Forrester, John, *The Seductions of Psychoanalysis: Freud, Lacan and Derrida*, Cambridge University Press, Cambridge, 1990.

Foucault, Michel, 'Madness, the Absence of Work', trans. Peter Stastny and Deniz Sengel, *Critical Inquiry*, vol. 21, Winter 1995, pp. 290–1.

Frazer, J. G., *The Golden Bough: A Study in Comparative Religions*, 2nd edn, Macmillan, London, 1900.

Freedheim, Donald K. (ed.), *History of Psychotherapy: A Century of Change*, American Psychological Association, Washington, D.C., 1992.

Freud, Sigmund, *The Interpretation of Dreams*, [1900], ed. Angela Richards, Penguin, London, 1991.

——, *Totem and Taboo: Some Points of Agreement Between the Mental Lives of Savages and Neurotics*, [1912–13], in *The Origins of Religion*, ed. and trans. James Strachey, Penguin, London, 1985, pp. 43–224.

——, 'Recollection, Repetition and Working Through', *Further Recommendations in the Technique of Psychoanalysis*, [1914], in *Freud: Therapy and Technique*, ed. Philip Rieff, Collier Books, New York, 1963.

——, 'Thoughts for the Times on War and Death', [1915], in *Civilisation, Society and Religion*, ed. Albert Dickson, Penguin, Harmondsworth, 1991, pp. 57–89.

——, *Beyond the Pleasure Principle*, [1920], in *On Metapsychology: The Theory of Psychoanalysis*, ed. Angela Richards, Penguin, Harmondsworth, 1985, pp. 269–338.

——, 'One of the Difficulties of Psycho-analysis', *International Journal of Psychoanalysis* vol. 1, no. 1, 1920, pp. 17–25.

——, *The Ego and the Id*, [1923], Norton, New York, 1960.

——, *The Ego and the Id*, [1923], in *Standard Edition XIX*, ed. and trans. James Strachey, The Hogarth Press, London, 1961.

——, *Civilization and its Discontents*, [1930], in *Civilisation, Society and Religion*, ed. Albert Dickson, Penguin, Harmondsworth, 1991, pp. 243–340.

——, 'The Dissection of the Psychical Personality', [1933], in *The Essentials of Psychoanalysis*, ed. Anna Freud, Penguin, London, 1986, pp. 484–504.

——, 'Analysis Terminable and Interminable', [1937], in *Freud: Therapy and Technique*, ed. Philip Rieff, Collier Books, New York, 1963.

——, *Moses and Monotheism*, [1939], in *The Origins of Religion*, ed. and trans. James Strachey, Penguin, London, 1985, pp. 237–386.

——, *Civilisation, Society and Religion*, ed. Albert Dickson, Penguin, Harmondsworth, 1991.

Frosh, Steven, *For and Against Psychoanalysis*, Routledge, London, 1997.

Gay, Peter, *Freud for Historians*, Oxford University Press, New York, 1985.

——, *The Naked Heart: The Bourgeois Experience, Victoria to Freud*, vol. IV, Fontana Press, London, 1998.

Gergen, Kenneth J., 'History and Psychology: Three Weddings and a Future', in Jan Lewis and Peter N. Stearns (eds), *An Emotional History of the United States*, New York University Press, New York, 1998, pp. 15–29.

Giddens, A., *The Transformation of Intimacy: Sexuality, Love and Eroticism in Modern Societies*, Polity, Cambridge, 1992.

Goldhagen, D., *Hitler's Willing Executioners*, Knopf, New York, 1996.

Goldstein, Jan (ed.), *Foucault and the Writing of History*, Blackwell, Oxford, 1994.

Green, Anna and Troup, Kathleen (eds), *The Houses of History: A Critical Reader in Twentieth-century History and Theory*, Manchester University Press, Manchester, 1999.

Grosz, Elizabeth, *Volatile Bodies: Toward a Corporeal Feminism*, Allen & Unwin, Sydney, 1994.

Halperin, David, *Saint Foucault: Towards a Gay Hagiography*, Oxford University Press, New York, 1995.

Harding, Celia, 'Making Sense of Sexuality', in C. Harding (ed.), *Sexuality: Psychoanalytic Perspectives*, Brunner-Routledge, Hove, 2001, pp. 1–17.

Held, David, *Models of Democracy*, Stanford University Press, Stanford, Calif., 1996.

Holmes, Richard, 'Biographer's Footsteps', *International Review of Psychoanalysis*, vol. 19, no. 1, 1992, pp. 1–8.

Horney, Karen, *Neurosis and Human Growth: The Struggle Toward Self-realisation*, W. W. Norton, New York, 1950.

Hunt, Lynn, 'No Longer an Evenly Flowing River: Time, History, and the Novel', *American Historical Review*, vol. 103, no. 5, December 1998, pp. 1517–21.

Isay, Richard A., *Becoming Gay: The Journey to Self-Acceptance*, Henry Holt, New York, 1996.

Jaanus, Maire, ' "A Civilisation of Hatred": The Other in the Imaginary', in Richard Feldstein, Bruce Fink and Maire Jaanus (eds), *Reading Seminars I and II: Lacan's Return to Freud*, State University of New York Press, Albany, 1996, pp. 323–55.

Jackson, Leonard, *Literature, Psychoanalysis and the New Sciences of the Mind*, Pearson, Essex, 2000.

Jones, Ernest, 'Editorial', *International Journal of Psycho-Analysis*, vol. 1, no. 1, 1920, pp. 3–7.

Klein, Hillel and Kogan, Ilany, 'Identification Processes and Denial in the Shadow of Nazism', *International Journal of Psycho-Analysis*, vol. 67, 1986, pp. 45–52.

Kohut, Heinz, *The Analysis of the Self*, International Universities Press, New York, 1971.

——, *The Restoration of the Self*, International Universities Press, New York 1977.

Kuklick, Henrika, *The Savage Within: The Social History of British Anthropology 1885–1945*, Cambridge University Press, Cambridge, 1991.

Kuper, Adam, *The Invention of Primitive Society: Transformations of an Illusion*, Routledge, London, 1988.

Lacan, Jacques, *The Four Fundamental Concepts of Psycho-Analysis*, ed. Jacques-Alain Miller, trans. Alan Sheridan, W. W. Norton, New York, 1981.

——, *The Ethics of Psychoanalysis 1959–1960*, The Seminar of Jacques Lacan, Book VII, ed. Jacques-Alain Miller, trans. Dennis Porter, Tavistock/Routledge, London 1992.

——, *On Feminine Sexuality: The Limits of Love and Knowledge*, The Seminar of Jacques Lacan, Book XX, ed. Jacques-Alain Miller, trans. Bruce Fink, W. W. Norton, New York, 1998.

LaCapra, Dominick, *Representing the Holocaust: History, Theory, Trauma*, Cornell University Press, Ithaca, N.Y., 1994.

——, *History and Memory After Auschwitz*, Cornell University Press, Ithaca, N.Y., 1998.

Laclau, Ernesto, 'The Death and Resurrection of the Theory of Ideology', *MLN*, vol. 112, no. 3, 1997, pp. 297–321.

La Nauze, J. A., *Alfred Deakin: A Biography*, 2 vols, Melbourne University Press, Melbourne, 1965.

Lane, Christopher, 'Psychoanalysis and Sexual Identity', in A. Medhurst and S. R. Munt (eds), *Lesbian and Gay Studies: A Critical Introduction*, Cassell, London, 1997, pp. 160–75.

Lasswell, Harold, *Psychopathology and Politics*, [1930], University of Chicago Press, Chicago, 1977.

Lee, Hermione, *Virginia Woolf*, Chatto & Windus, London, 1996.

Lefebvre, Henri, *The Production of Space*, trans. Donald Nicholson-Smith, Blackwell, Oxford 1991.

Levenson, Michael H., *A Genealogy of Modernism: A Study of English Literary Doctrine 1908–1922*, Cambridge University Press, Cambridge, 1984.

Lewis, Jan and Stearns, Peter N. (eds), *An Emotional History of the United States*, New York University Press, New York, 1998.

Likierman, Meira, *Melanie Klein: Her Work in Context*, Continuum, London, 2001.

Little, Graham, 'The Uses of Childhood', *Eureka Street*, September 1994, pp. 28–32.

Lunbeck, Elizabeth, *The Psychiatric Persuasion: Knowledge, Gender and Power in Modern America*, Princeton University Press, Princeton, N.J., 1994.

MacKenzie, S. P., 'Prisoners of War and Civilian Internees: The Asian and Pacific Theatres', in Loyd E. Lee (ed.), *World War II in Asia and the Pacific and the War's Aftermath, with General Themes: A Handbook of Literature and Research*, Greenwood Press, Westport, Conn., 1998, pp. 172–82.

McLaren, Angus, *Twentieth-Century Sexuality: A History*, Blackwell, London, 1999.

McLeary, Ailsa with Dingle, Tony, *Catherine: On Catherine Currie's Diary, 1878–1908*, Melbourne University Press, Melbourne, 1998.

McLennan, John Ferguson, *Primitive Marriage: An Inquiry into the Origin of the Form of Capture in Marriage Ceremonies*, [1865], ed. Peter Riviere, University of Chicago Press, Chicago, Ill., 1970.

March, Cristie, 'Crimson Silks and New Potatoes: The Heteroglossic Power of the Object in Atwood's *Alias Grace*', *Studies in Canadian Literature*, vol. 22, no. 1, 1997, pp. 66–82.

Masson, Jeffrey, *The Assault on Truth: Freud's Suppression of the Seduction Theory*, Faber, London, 1984.

Micale, Mark, 'Paradigm and Ideology in Psychiatric History Writing: The Case of Psychoanalysis', in *Journal of Nervous and Mental Disease*, vol. 184, 1996, pp. 146–52.

Micale, Mark and Lerner, Paul (eds), *Traumatic Pasts: History, Psychiatry, Trauma and the Modern Age, 1870–1930*, Cambridge University Press, Cambridge, 2001.

Mills, James H., *Madness, Cannabis and Colonialism: The 'Native Only' Lunatic Asylums of British India, 1857–1900*, St. Martin's Press, New York, 2000.

Mitchell, Juliet (ed.), *The Selected Melanie Klein*, Penguin, London, 1986.

Morgan, Kenneth O., 'Writing Political Biography', in Eric Hamburger and John Charley (eds), *The Troubled Face of Biography*, Macmillan, London, 1988.

Morgan, Lewis Henry, *Ancient Society*, [1877], ed. Leslie A White, Belknap Press of Harvard University Press, Cambridge, Mass., 1964.

Morrison, Toni, *Beloved*, Picador, London, 1987.

National Archives of Australia, CRS A1, 1938/33269; CRS A452, 1954/575; CRS A659, 1939/1/5250.

O'Carroll, Larry, 'Against the Grain: When Gay Men Counsel Other Gay Men', *Psychodynamic Counselling*, vol. 5, no. 1, 1999, pp. 25–51.

O'Connor, Noreen and Ryan, Joanna, *Wild Desires and Mistaken Identities: Lesbianism and Psychoanalysis*, Virago, London, 1993.

O'Loughlin, M., 'Education for Citizenship: Integrating Knowledge, Imagination and Democratic Dispositions', *Forum of Education: A Journal of Theory, Research, Policy and Practice*, vol. 52, no. 2, November 1997, pp. 24–33.

Ong, Walter J., *Orality and Literacy: The Technologizing of the Word*, Methuen, London, 1982.

Otero, Francisco and Escardo, Adela, 'Sexuality in the Age of AIDS', *International Journal of Psycho-analysis*, vol. 79, no. 1, 1998, pp. 136–9.

Pascal, Blaise, 'Le Coeur a ses Raisons que la Raison ne Connoist Point' in *Pascal's Pensees*, trans. H. F. Stewart, Pantheon Books, New York, 1950.

Pateman, Carole, *The Sexual Contract*, Polity Press, Cambridge, 1988.

Peterson, Nicolas, 'Donald Thomson: A Biographical Sketch', in *Donald Thomson in Arnhem Land*, Curry O'Neill Ross, Melbourne, 1983, pp. 1–15.

Pfister, Joel and Schnog, Nancy (eds), *Inventing the Psychological: Toward a Cultural History of Emotional Life in America*, Yale University Press, New Haven, Conn., 1997.

Phillips, Adam, *Terrors and Experts*, Faber & Faber, London, 1995/1997.

——, *Promises, Promises: Essays on Literature and Psychoanalysis*, Faber & Faber, London, 2000.

Pick, Daniel, 'Freud's Group Psychology and the History of the Crowd', *History Workshop Journal*, no. 40, Autumn 1995, pp. 30–61.

Piddington, Marion, *Tell Them! or The Second Stage of Mothercraft*, Moore's Bookshop, Sydney, 1926.

Porter, Laurence M., *The Interpretation of Dreams: Freud's Theories Revisited*, Twayne Publishers, Boston, 1987.

Porter, Roy, *A Social History of Madness: The World Through the Eyes of the Insane*, Weidenfeld & Nicholson, New York, 1988.

Pound, Ezra, 'The Tradition', [1913], in T. S. Eliot (ed.), *Literary Essays by Ezra Pound*, New Directions, New York, 1968.

Ramet, Sabrina, *Balkan Babel: The Disintegration of Yugoslavia from the Death of Tito to Ethnic War*, Westview Press, Boulder, Colo., 1996.

Read, Peter, *Returning to Nothing: The Meaning of Lost Places*, Cambridge University Press, Cambridge, 1996.

Reeson, Margaret, *A Very Long War*, Melbourne University Press, Melbourne, 2000.

Reiger, Kerreen M., *The Disenchantment of the Home: Modernising the Australian Family 1880–1940*, Oxford University Press, Melbourne, 1985.

Reynolds, Robert, *Remaking the Homosexual: From Camp to Queer*, Melbourne University Press, Melbourne, 2002.

Rickard, John, *H. B. Higgins: The Rebel as Judge*, George Allen & Unwin, Sydney, 1984.

——, *A Family Romance: The Deakins at Home*, Melbourne University Press, Melbourne, 1996.

Rogerson, Margaret, 'Reading the Patchworks in *Alias Grace*', *The Journal of Commonwealth Literature*, vol. 33, no. 1, 1998, pp. 5–22.

Roper, Lyndal, *Oedipus and the Devil: Witchcraft, Sexuality and Religion in Early Modern Europe*, Routledge, London, 1994.

Rorty, R., *Contingency, Irony and Solidarity*, Cambridge University Press, Cambridge, 1989.

Rose, Nikolas, *Inventing Ourselves: Psychology, Power and Personhood*, Cambridge University Press, Cambridge, 1996.

Rousseau, Jean-Jacques, 'A Discourse on the Origins of Inequality', in *The Social Contract and the Discourses*, rev. ed., trans. G. D. H. Cole, Everyman's Library, London, 1973, pp. 31–125.

Royston, Robert, 'Sexuality and Object Relations', in C. Harding (ed.), *Sexuality: Psychoanalytic Perspectives*, Brunner-Routledge, Hove, 2001, pp. 35–51.

Rubin, Gayle, 'Sexual Traffic: Gayle Rubin Interviewed by Judith Butler', in M. Merk et al. (eds), *Coming Out of Feminism*, Blackwell, Oxford, pp. 36–73.

Russell, Denise, *Women, Madness and Medicine*, Polity, Cambridge, Mass., 1995.

Ryan, Judith, *The Vanishing Subject: Early Psychology and Literary Modernism*, University of Chicago Press, Chicago, Ill., 1991.

Sadkovich, James J., *The U.S. Media and Yugoslavia: 1991–1995*, Praeger, Westport, Conn., 1998.

Schwartz, Joseph, *Cassandra's Daughter: A History of Psychoanalysis in Europe and America*, Penguin/Allen Lane, London, 1999.

Smith, Bernard, *Modernism's History: A Study in Twentieth-century Art and Ideas*, UNSW Press, Sydney, 1998.

Stallybrass, Peter and White, Allon, *The Politics and Poetics of Transgression*, Cornell University Press, Ithaca, N.Y., 1986.

Steele, Jeffrey, 'The Gender and Racial Politics of Mourning in Antebellum America', in Jan Lewis and Peter N. Stearns (eds), *An Emotional History of the United States*, New York University Press, New York, 1998, pp. 91–106.

Still, Arthur and Velody, Irving (eds), *Rewriting the History of Madness: Studies in Foucault's* Histoire de la folie, Routledge, London, 1992.

Stocking, George W., *Victorian Anthropology*, The Free Press, London, 1982.

Strachey, Lytton, *Eminent Victorians*, Chatto & Windus, London, 1918.

Strozier, Charles B., *Heinz Kohut: The Making of a Psychoanalyst*, Farrar, Strauss & Giroux, New York, 2001.

Tal, Kali, *World(s) of Hurt: Reading the Literature of Trauma*, Cambridge University Press, Cambridge, 1996.

Theweleit, Klaus, *Male Fantasies*, vol. 1, University of Minnesota Press, Minneapolis, Minn., 1987.

Thomson, Donald, Papers, Melbourne Museum.

——, Private Papers, held by Mrs Dorita Thomson.

——, Interim General Report of Preliminary Expedition to Arnhem Land, Northern Territory of Australia, 1935–36, NAA, CRS A52, 572/994THO.

——, Recommendations of Policy in Native Affairs in the Northern Territory of Australia, *Commonwealth Parliamentary Papers*, 1937–40, vol. III.

——, *Report on Expedition to Arnhem Land, 1936–37*, Government Printer, Canberra, 1939.

——, *'Justice' for Aborigines*, Herald, Melbourne, 1947.

——, *Donald Thomson in Arnhem Land*, comp. and introduced by Nicolas Peterson, Currey O'Neill Ross, Melbourne, 1983.

Thomson of Arnhem Land, dir. John Moore, Film Australia/John Moore Productions, Sydney, 2000.

Thompson, Mark, *Forging War: The Media in Serbia, Croatia and Bosnia–Herzegovina*, Article 19, London, 1994.

Tucker, Robert C., 'A Stalin Biographer's Memoir', in Samuel Baron and Carl Pletsch (eds), *Introspection in Biography: The Biographer's Quest for Self-awareness*, Analytic Press, Hillsdale, N.J., 1985, pp. 249–71.

Tylor, Edward Burnett, *Primitive Culture: Researches into the Development of Mythology, Philosophy, Religion, Language, Art and Custom*, 2 vols, John Murray, London, 1891.

valentine, kylie, The Making of Modern Madness: British Modernism, Psychoanalysis and Psychiatry between the Wars, PhD, University of Sydney, 1999.

Walter, James, *The Leader: A Political Biography*, University of Queensland Press, St Lucia, Qld, 1980.

Waterford, Van, *Prisoners of the Japanese in World War II*, McFarland & Co., Jefferson, N.C., 1994.

Weiner, Dora B., 'Esquirol's Patient Register: The First Private Psychiatric Hospital in Paris, 1802–1808', *Bulletin of the History of Medicine*, vol. 63, 1989, pp. 110–20.

Weiss, Gail, *Body Images: Embodiment as Intercorporeality*, Routledge, London, 1999.

White, Richard, *Inventing Australia: Images and Identity 1788–1980*, Allen & Unwin, Sydney, 1981.

Whitebook, Joel, *Perversion and Utopia. A Study in Psychoanalysis and Critical Theory*, MIT Press, Cambridge, Mass., 1995.

Winnicott, Donald, *Home Is Where We Start From*, Penguin, Harmondsworth, 1950.

——, *Through Paediatrics to Psycho-analysis*, Hogarth, London, 1951.

Wolfe, Patrick, 'On Being Woken Up: The Dreamtime in Anthropology and in Australian Settler Culture', *Comparative Studies in Society and History*, vol. 33, 1991, pp. 197–224.

Woolf, Virginia, *Mrs Dalloway*, [1925], Hogarth Press, London, 1958.

Wrong, D., *Skeptical Sociology*, Columbia University Press, New York, 1976.

Zaretsky, Eli, 'Identity Theory, Identity Politics: Psychoanalysis, Marxism, Post-Structuralism', in C. Calhoun (ed.), *Social Theory and the Politics of Identity*, Blackwell, Oxford, 1994, pp. 198–215.

Zizek, Slavoj, *The Plague of Fantasies*, Verso, London, 1997.

——, *The Ticklish Subject*, Verso, London, 1999.

Journals

Angry Penguins

Australasian Journal of Psychology and Philosophy

Australasian Nurses' Journal

Everylady's Journal

Mankind

Medical Journal of Australia

Women's World

Index

Abelove, Henry, 51, 52
abjection, 111; and gender, 109
Aboriginality: and Aboriginal dreaming, 31; and Aboriginal rights in Australia, 8, 96–105; and assimilationism, 97, 101, 103, 105; and attitudes to mixed races, 104; and Indigenous Australians, 60–70, 99–105, 139; othering of, 98; and segregation, 101, 102–3
Adorno, Theodor, 194
adultery, 33
Age newspaper, 20
aggression, 69, 70
Alexander, Sally, 3, 17, 19
Althusser, Louis, 194–5, 196
Altman, Dennis, 10, 55
ambivalence: historians' use of, 157; and psychoanalysis, 7
American Psychoanalytic Association, 52
American Revolution, 129
Amiel, Henri-Frédéric, 9, 107, 111–16
ancient hatreds thesis, 141–52
Anderson, Benedict, 128
Anderson, Perry, 38, 41
anthropology, 3, 69; and evolutionary theory, 98; and Freud, 5, 66–70; history of, 5, 64; and postcolonialism, 97; and psycho-analysis, 60, 106; and study of Aboriginal culture, 97
anti-Semitism, 192; *see also* Holocaust
Arakun, 99, 100, 101
Aristotle, 127, 133
Assembly of Citizens of Serbian Nationality and of Serb Ethnic Origin of Bosnia, 148
Atlantic Charter, 103

attachment, 10, 133–5; and national identity, 130, 136–40; and place, 130, 136–40
Attwood, Bain, 8, 96–105
Atwood, Margaret, *Alias Grace*, 12, 177–87
Australian Aborigines' League, 96
Australian and New Zealand Association, 159
Australian Army Medical Corps, 28
Australian culture: and anti-intellectualism, 124–5; and colonial work ethic, 125; and fairness, 125; and gender relations, 128; and race relations, 128; and religion, 122–3; and the social imaginary, 128–9; *see also* nationalism, and Australian identity
Australian intellectuals, 4, 27, 28, 30, 31, 35
Australian National Research Council (ANRC), 98, 207n
Austro-Hungarian Empire, 142

Baker, Bettina, 159
Bakhtin, Mikhail, 110
Balibar, Etiene, 150–1
Balkan Wars, 141; historical narratives of, 142, 143
Balkan tribalism, 10, 141, 147, 149, 150; as social fantasy, 142, 144
Barker, Philip, 63
Baumann, Zygmut, 32
belonging, *see* attachment
Benjamin, Jessica, 188–9
Berkeley, George, 40
Bersani, Leo, 49
Bieber, Irving, 52
bigamy, 33
biography: *Australian Dictionary of Biography*, 93; and history, 84–95; literary, 74; politi-

226

dream analysis, 4, 31, 33–4, 85–7; and anxiety, 33; history of, 33; reading history through, 33; and the self, 32–3
dreams, 6, 27; Freud on, 68–9; history of, 26–35
drives, 7, 8, 50, 56, 79; Freud on, 76; and Lacanian theory, 167
Duguid, Charles, 100

Edel, Leon, 74, 82–3
ego, 4, 12, 69–70, 107; bodily, 107–11; historical specificity of, 108–9; ideal, 134
ego psychology, 14, 52, 120
electro-shock therapy, 159
Elias, Norbert, 111
Eliot, T. S., 43
Elkin, A. P., 31
Elliot, Anthony, 135
Elster, John, 188
embodiment, 3, 37, 46; and the body politic, 110; and gender, 109, 111–16; and health, 107–16; history of, 107; and history of manners, 111; libidinal investment in, 108–9, 111; and morality, 107–8, 111, 112, 115; in nineteenth century, 111–16; and object-relations theory, 133; and place, 130–1, 138–40; *see also* body; interiority/exteriority
emotion, 8, 14, 33–4, 58, 79–80, 133–4, 191; grammar of, 7, 55, 80; history of, 3, 35; management of, 32; in object relations, 134–5; and structures of feeling, 106; *see also* Klein, Melanie
empathy, psychology and politics of, 8
Encyclopaedia Britannica, 65
English Civil War, 124
English Revolution, 129
Enlightenment, 62, 191
Erikson, Erik, 10, 13, 14, 74, 120; *Childhood and Society*, 193; on the ego, 120–1, 122; and Freudian theory, 121, 125; on identification, 121; on identity, 14, 119, 120; on identity crisis, 120; on interiority/exteriority, 120–1; on socialisation, 122, 127, 193–5; *Young Man Luther*, 76
Eros, Freud on, 178
ethnicity, 14; ethnic cleansing, 147, 151; and homogeneity, 148–51; *see also* nationalism, and ethnicity
eugenics, 29; and race, 29–30
European Commission, 144–5, 149
European philosophical tradition, 10, 133
Everylady's Journal, 30
evolutionary theory, 43, 64, 65
exogamy, 65

exteriority, *see* interiority/exteriority

Fabian, Johannes, 67
fantasy, 5, 50, 60, 191, 198; aggressive, 13; of ancient hatred, 141–52; and anxiety, 143; Freud on, 42, 43; and history, 190; ideological nature of, 142, 143; individual and collective, 111, 135, 142; and national identity, 130, 132, 135, 141–52; and sexuality, 32, 58–9; social forms of, 10; unconscious, 48, 128, 190
fascism, 175, 194
Faye, Esther, 11, 12, 166–76
Feher, Michael, 145, 148–9, 152
Fein, Yvonne, 11, 167–76, 214n
feminism: feminist criticism, 44; and Freudian theory, 29; and motherhood, 29; and psychoanalysis, 3; second-wave, 124
feminist historians, 3
fetishism, 65
Figlio, Karl, 3
Fison, Lorimer, 66
fisting, 57–9
Fitzpatrick, Brian, 103
Forgioni, Stella, 160
Forrester, John, 42
Forth, Christopher E., 2, 8, 106–16
Foucault, Michel, 8,18, 57; on archaeology, 19; on body and subjectivity, 108; influence of, 49, 55–6; on madness, 24; and psychoanalysis, 56; and repressive hypothesis, 56; on the subject, 53
Fouché, Joseph, 84
Frankfurt School, and psychoanalysis, 191–2
Frazer, Sir James, 65
free association, 8, 29, 87
French Revolution, 84, 129
Freud, Anna, 173
Freud, Sigmund, 13, 21, 37, 49, 79, 82, 84, 168, 190, 195, 212n; 'Analysis Terminable and Interminable', 178, 179; and anthropology, 5, 66–70; *Beyond the Pleasure Principle*, 178; on childhood, 80–1; *Civilisation and its Discontents*, 39; on death drive, 174, 178; on desire, 52, 61; 'The Dissection of the Psychical Personality', 69; on dreams, 52, 61; on drives, 76; *The Ego and the Id*, 108; on ego and superego, 2; on Eros, 178; on fantasy, 42, 43; *The Future of an Illusion*, 39; on group psychology, 4; 'Group Psychology and the Analysis of the Ego', 194, 197; on heterosexuality, 51; and history, 42; on homosexuality, 5, 51–2; on identity, 66; *The Interpretation of Dreams*, 31, 181; on masochism, 173; on memory, 4, 44; *Moses*